STAY *with* ME

STAY

with ME

STORIES OF A
BLACK BAG DOCTOR

To Jeawell

with blessings

Judy Pickard

ANDERSON SPICKARD JR., MD
WITH BARBARA R. THOMPSON

ISBN-10 1-4609-1378-7
ISBN-13 978-1-4609-1378-9
LCCN 2011902584

To Sue,

who made it all possible

The friend who can be silent with us in a moment of despair and confusion, who can stay with us in an hour of grief and bereavement, who can tolerate not knowing, not curing, not healing, and face with us the reality of our powerlessness, that is a friend who cares.

—Henri Nouwen

CONTENTS

ACKNOWLEDGMENTS

We need to be angels for each other, to give each other strength and consolation. Because only when we fully realize that the cup of life is not only a cup of sorrow but also a cup of joy will we be able to drink it.

—Henri Nouwen

I want to express my heartfelt gratitude to those with whom I have been privileged to share my professional and personal life journey. To name them all would require another book, but I am especially indebted to:

Sue Spickard, for our fifty-two years together and in celebration of our three children and eleven grandchildren. Sue has been the courageous, honest, and down-to-earth center of the storm throughout our marriage, and her work in nonprofits and church programs has touched the lives of many.

My teachers and colleagues at Vanderbilt Medical School and Hospital, who, through their personal care for patients and myriad conferences and lectures, helped me forge the skills of diagnosis and treatment: Josh Billings, Amos Christie, Bill Hillman, Grant Liddle, David Rogers, Bill Scott, John Shapiro, Jud Randolph, and others. Over the years, many colleagues gave friendship and help in diagnosing and treating difficult patients, including John Oates, Glenn Koenig, Dewey Dunn, John Griscom, Oscar Crofford, Bud Friesinger, Frank Gluck, Craig Heim, Allen Kaiser, John Leonard, John Sergent, and Sheldon Wolfe. Clifton Meador, whose own books provide a humorous and fascinating glimpse into the practice of medicine, deserves a special note of gratitude for kindly writing the preface to *Stay with Me*.

Lee Cluff and Frank Iber at Johns Hopkins; Vernon Knight and Jack Utz at the National Institutes of Health.

Ruby Hearn and Paul Jellinek, for our work together with the Robert Wood Johnson Foundation Fighting Back program, and to Greg Dixon, whose friendship, wisdom, and humor have been one of life's great gifts.

Bill Swiggart and Ron Neufeld, who are not only treasured colleagues but friends and have provided stable leadership and wisdom for many years to the Vanderbilt Institute for Treatment of Addiction (VITA). We are all indebted to Peter Martin, MD, for his psychiatric support of VITA and extensive knowledge of addiction and comorbid psychiatric illnesses. I am also grateful to Charlene Dewey, MD, MEd, who along with Bill is bringing visionary energy to the Center for Professional Health.

To Lucille Aydelott, Carolyn Sanders, and Diana Phillips. We worked together in my Vanderbilt offices for a span of over forty years, and without their dedicated and capable assistance, my work would have been impossible.

To wise spiritual teachers who enriched my faith journey immeasurably: Walter Courtney, Mark DeVries, Heine and Agnes Germann Edey, Norman Grubb, and Jim Kitchen.

To Howell and Madeline Adams, and Alfred and Carney Farris, who have inspired me and helped me stay grounded since our college years together; their life work has made the world a far better place. Among many other philanthropic legacies, Howell and Madeline funded the Anderson Spickard, Jr., Chancellor's Chair in Medicine at Vanderbilt Medical Center. Alfred and Carney have enriched the lives of countless people as organic farmers and long-term friends of the Soroti region of Uganda. As we move together into new roles as elders and "keepers of the meaning," our friendships remain one of life's great treasures.

Finally, Barbara Thompson and I have worked together for almost three decades, writing and thinking about addiction. Her writing skills and insights into the human condition have been enriched by her work with survivors of war. Most recently, she has helped found the Global Village School for refugee teen girls in Decatur, Georgia. I am profoundly grateful for our collaboration and friendship.

Note: Names and details have been changed to
protect the privacy of individuals.

PREFACE

Andy Spickard's stories, in *Stay with Me*, capture the flavor and spirit of an era in clinical medicine that will never come again. We begin our journey with him in medical school. We are there on the Osler Service at Johns Hopkins, when he struggles as a new resident to keep alive an alcoholic patient dying from heatstroke, acute diabetes, and bleeding esophageal varices. We are drawn into the hectic life of the medical house staff in the days when there was no such thing as time off and no maximum eighty-hour workweek for residents. Spickard carries us with him through those unrelenting nights of twenty-four-hour call.

We follow Spickard in private practice as he treats a botulism patient in an iron lung, reminding us of the days before ventilators were invented. He uncovers a "Typhoid Mary," treats tapeworm and rare fungus disease, and invents a warning mechanism to save young athletes from heatstroke. We see him making house calls to patients too ill to come to the office. Sometimes, when the patient is far beyond curative medical care, he has nothing more to offer than his own presence.

And then the writing shifts gears. Spickard is introduced to the mysteries of alcohol addiction through the drive to understand the denial and cravings of alcoholic patients. He adopts as his life mission the task of creating a national and international movement to understand and treat alcoholism. He and Barbara Thompson write the classic book on addicted drinking, *Dying for a Drink*, and it is translated into multiple languages, including Russian and Mongolian.

Meanwhile, Spickard creates a national program to make sure alcohol addiction is added to the curriculum of every medical school in the United States, helping establish it as a disease understood to be fatal if not treated. He takes his ideas and energy to Russia, where alcohol has lowered the life expectancy of males to less than sixty years. We meet Russians struggling to bring Alcoholics Anonymous and Twelve Step spirituality into treatment programs.

Until the end of his career, Spickard remains the quintessential doctor, a medical professional who, while retaining close and intimate contact with his patients, is able to remain emotionally detached. Then comes retirement, with its insomnia, anxieties, and depression, and a deep, dark doubt that anyone could ever understand him as a person.

At an Alcoholics Anonymous meeting for visitors, Spickard is finally able to reach out for personal help, reminding us of the wounded healer in each one of us. He finds a spiritual home in Alcoholics Anonymous, not from any personal addiction, but from the joy of connecting with other suffering humans who are willing to share their lives with one another.

This is a powerful and well-written book about medicine at its deepest level of healing. I hope that it will be read not only by laypeople but by every medical student and every physician, young and old. Spickard's story is our own history, and it will help us pass on, from one generation to the next, the blessings, challenges, and privileges of practicing medicine.

Clifton J. Meador, MD
Professor of Medicine
Vanderbilt Medical Center

INTRODUCTION

Stay with me.

This poignant appeal by Jesus, spoken to his closest friends on the night before his death, has profound meaning for me, as a person and a doctor. I have said the same words to patients who are losing consciousness. I have heard them from patients during critical or even routine illnesses. They are the words I myself spoke to friends and family during my own dark hour.

The stories in *Stay with Me* come from my fifty years of medical practice as a "black bag doctor," a physician who is willing to make house calls. In many ways, they are dispatches from an era of medical practice that, in the twenty-first century, is rapidly disappearing. A patient surviving botulism with the help of an iron lung. A chronic alcoholic trapped in a horsehair chair. The desperate ride in an ambulance with a patient bleeding to death. In the end, they are all lessons in *staying with* patients as they make the journey from poor health to recovery, or learn to live with a chronic illness, or face impending death.

My own journey in medicine began long before I entered medical school. Like many doctors of my era, I was an oldest son and a "caretaker" growing up. When I was eighteen, my father was struck and killed by lightning while he was playing golf. His good cheer and wisdom had guided me all my life, and I could not imagine how my family and I were going to continue our lives without him. Except for the support of my mother and two sisters, our closely knit extended family, and caring friends, I'm not sure how I would have made it through this ordeal.

My father's death reinforced my determination to study medicine. After medical school and an internship at Vanderbilt, I did additional training and research in infectious diseases at Johns Hopkins and the National Institutes of Health. In the mid-'60s, I returned to Nashville where I trained as a specialist in infectious disease, entered private practice medicine, and began teaching at Vanderbilt. I have remained there ever since.

Through it all, I was fortunate to train with a series of highly qualified mentors. They taught me the art and science of medicine, and how to distinguish the gravely ill from the sick or the worried well. I learned to listen carefully to a patient's history, give a thorough physical, separate the meaningful from the trivial, and deduce my way to a proper diagnosis and best course of treatment.

What I wasn't taught was how to identify and deal with the murky waters of emotional illness and addiction. Although we learned as students that 40 percent of our patients' illnesses were of psychosomatic origin, we didn't learn how to talk with them about their emotional or spiritual lives. I learned to recognize and detoxify a late-stage alcoholic but not how to identify or treat earlier stages of addiction. Addicts who came to my office left without getting the life-saving help they needed.

In the 1970s, I was asked to be a consulting physician in the case of a brilliant young doctor who was pouring large amounts of pure ethanol into his Coca-Cola. He was a friend as well as a colleague, and he listened with openness and embarrassment as I reminded him of the serious health consequences of heavy drinking. He agreed to cut back and go to meetings of Alcoholics Anonymous. Instead, he kept drinking, and a few weeks later he shot himself.

I was baffled and sick at heart. What could I have done differently? Was there a protocol for treating addiction that I hadn't heard about? In medicine, not to know the right treatment is a major failing, but to think you know when you don't know is even worse.

My search for information took me to St. Mary's Hospital in Minnesota. There I experienced firsthand a groundbreaking and successful treatment program that combined medical science with the program of Alcoholics Anonymous. The Twelve Steps resonated with my own Christian spirituality, and because of AA's nonsectarian approach, I knew it would also be acceptable to my medical colleagues.

I thought I had found the Holy Grail of medicine. I began to recognize addiction when I saw it, and I directed my patients to treatment programs and Alcoholics Anonymous. I expanded my focus to include other addictions, community prevention programs, and even impaired and/or disruptive physicians. I wrote *Dying for a Drink* with Barbara R. Thompson. After this book was translated into Russian, among other languages, I made two trips to Moscow. I witnessed the country's catastrophic drinking problem and met with leaders of their fledgling AA movement.

> In a culture that generally celebrates empowerment and self-esteem, A.A. begins with disempowerment. The goal is to get people to gain control over their lives, but it all begins with an act of surrender and an admission of weakness.
>
> —David Brooks
> *The New York Times*

My work with addicted patients and my firsthand experience of the miracle of recovery have given me enormous professional and personal satisfaction. Like many other people without a personal experience of addiction, I feel that I owe much to the Twelve Steps of Alcoholics Anonymous. In particular, I am drawn to the Third Step: *Made a decision to turn our will and our lives over to the care of God as we understood Him.* I made that decision in 1973, and now Jesus and the Holy Spirit are my life. Their life in me has given me power to pray in faith for those caught in the web of addiction. I trust God to lead me, and for this I will be thankful forever.

After my retirement in 2008, I fell into a depression that was complicated by a painful physical illness. It was my turn to ask family and friends to "stay with me." I will always be grateful to them and to the community of Alcoholics Anonymous, which continued to embrace me in a dark and incomprehensible hour. They are among the people with whom I have shared the joys and sorrows of life, its terror and consolations, and I cannot thank them enough.

Anderson Spickard Jr., MD

1

QUEEN OF THE GYPSIES

The fifty-year-old woman with long dark hair was lying on a gurney, her eyes and skin turning yellow. Her name was Angela, and she had been sick for a week with fever. She had red spots on her chest, and she had arrived an hour earlier at the hospital complaining of a serious pain in her upper right side. A nurse quietly explained to me that Angela was queen of the Roma Gypsies in East Tennessee.

After my second year of medical school, to get some practical experience, I was spending the summer as an extern on a surgical service of St. Mary's in Kingsport, Tennessee. I wrote orders for incoming patients who were then admitted to the care of senior surgeons. The attending physician, Dr. Gary Simmonds, assigned me to take Angela's history and give her an exam. I was the lowest person on the list of her caretakers, but the nurses called me doctor, and Angela didn't know otherwise. She was "my" patient, and I did my best to look like I knew what I was doing.*

---

* I also served as "first assistant" in surgery, where I learned to use retractors and a Bovie cautery to stop the bleeding of small blood vessels. My role was not unusual in a small community hospital because there were no residents to act as junior support to the senior staff. I had similar luck the next year at the Children's Hospital in Boston, where I scrubbed in on complex heart surgery.

The simple task of taking Angela's history, however, proved far more complicated than I expected. The Roma queen was morbidly obese. She was also surrounded by a large group of supporters. Like Angela, the women had dark hair and wore brightly colored skirts. The men were dressed in dark coats and white shirts. Every time I asked Angela a question, her royal retinue chimed in all together. It was impossible to understand a word that they were saying.

Finally, I sent everyone out of the room, except for two family members. They described Angela's symptoms in great detail and spoke admiringly of her legendary appetite. I took painstaking notes and ordered lab work, which confirmed that Angela had jaundice and a serious infection in her gallbladder and liver. Even with just two years of medical school, I knew that she needed immediate surgery. A diseased gallbladder that is not quickly removed can perforate, causing bile to spill into the abdomen and creating a widespread, life-threatening infection.

I admitted Angela to the hospital and called Dr. Simmonds. He came within minutes and scheduled Angela for emergency surgery to remove her gallbladder and any gallstones. Meanwhile, the nurse asked the Gypsies in the hall to leave, so they took up residence in the stairwell and spilled down all seven levels to the lobby. At the nurse's request, Dr. Simmonds tried to explain to them that they were violating the hospital's fire code. After a great deal of arguing back and forth, the group agreed to go home until Angela's early morning surgery.

When I came back to check on Angela later that evening, however, I could still hear the Gypsies in the stairwell. Their continuous low moaning sounded like a Greek chorus anticipating a tragedy. *If they are praying for me,* I remember thinking, *it's a good idea.* I was young and inexperienced, and I was about to be the first assistant on their queen's operation. At Vanderbilt, a lowly medical student like me would never have served in such a critical position; the opportunity would have gone to a resident. The most I could have hoped for was retractor duty, holding back the sides of an incision so that the surgeon could see what he or she was doing. The chance to play a significant role in Angela's surgery was a dream come true.

By the next morning, the moaning in the stairwell had reached new levels of pathos and urgency. We took Angela to the operating room with a dirgelike hum ringing in our ears. When Dr. Simmonds made his incision, fluid immediately rose from Angela's inflamed liver and gallbladder. The walls of her gallbladder were dangerously thin, but it had not yet ruptured.

Inside the gallbladder, we found a large stone that was forcing bile to back up in the liver. Normally, with the stone removed, her bile duct would drain properly, and her liver would return to health. But Angela's massive obesity made any operation hazardous. The list of potential problems was long and frightening: pneumonia, heart failure, a blood clot traveling from her large and motionless legs to her lungs, and a host of other complications found in obese patients.

Nonetheless, the surgery went well. When the incision was closed, we gave Angela intravenous antibiotics and put drains in her wound to take care of the postsurgery accumulation of fluids. Afterward, to avoid the Gypsies in the stairwell, we took the elevator down to the waiting room to speak with her immediate family. They were relieved to hear that Angela didn't have cancer.

"Angela is in critical condition because of her obesity and inflamed liver," Dr. Simmonds explained. "But barring any unforeseen complications, we expect her to make a complete recovery." The happy news spread quickly to the Gypsies in the stairwell. Their moaning stopped, and jubilant shouts echoed on every floor of the hospital. People crowded into the waiting room to congratulate the medical team.

Unfortunately, within twenty-four hours, it was clear that Angela was in serious trouble. For reasons that we could not determine, her liver continued to fail and her jaundice worsened. The Gypsies again took over the stairway and filled the hospital corridors with their mournful cries. Angela's family members kept a bedside vigil in her room. I checked on Angela continually, but she was barely responsive and stared vacantly around her room. Hospitals at that time did not have intensive care units, and by today's standards, even our recovery rooms were primitive. There was little that we could do except withhold food until her stomach could tolerate it.

The third night after surgery, I received an emergency call. Angela's family members had reported that she was not breathing. By the time I arrived, the queen of the East Tennessee Gypsies had died, and Dr. Simmonds was pronouncing her dead.

I watched Dr. Simmonds carefully while he delivered the sad news to the family. In medical school, I had not been trained (nor would I ever be) to tell family members that someone they loved had died. I knew I had to learn this skill by observation. As more and more Gypsies crowded into the room, Dr. Simmonds calmly explained that Angela most likely had died from a heart attack or a pulmonary embolus. Her friends and family received this news with heartrending cries of grief and sorrow. I knew nothing about the Roma, but I understood that for them the death of Angela was a great historical event, like the passing of a president.

Dr. Simmonds asked Angela's immediate family to give permission for a postmortem, so that we could determine the exact cause of death and perhaps prevent the deaths of other patients with her symptoms. A postmortem is a hard sell to any stunned and grieving family, and, not surprisingly, Angela's family adamantly refused. Minutes later, a group of Gypsies arrived in the room pushing a gurney. They loaded up the queen's body and wheeled it out of the room.

I watched from a window on the seventh floor as the Gypsies carefully placed the body of their queen into the back of a long white hearse. The hearse slowly pulled away, followed by an entourage of thirty or forty cars. It was the last I saw of the East Tennessee Gypsies. To this day, I wonder what kind of celebration we might have experienced if Queen Angela had survived her operation.

2

FIRST HOUSE CALL:
A DEATH IN THE FAMILY

The setting for my first house call could not have been more tranquil. It was a hot and muggy day as I pulled into the family farm of the grandparents of my cousin, Chris. Chris's grandfather, Jesse, had worked his small farm with his wife for over fifty years. Jesse had always been a good farmer, and the old barn where Chris and I had played in the hay as children was still standing. Rain barrels stood under each gutter to catch water for the kitchen garden and an abundant crop of summer vegetables.

Chris had called me less than an hour earlier. I was in the middle of seeing patients at my new office in the Medical Arts Building next door to Vanderbilt Hospital. I had only recently entered into private practice in internal medicine with my two partners, Josh Billings and John Griscom, who were far more experienced than I was.

"Andy, I need you to come right now," Chris said. "Jesse has shot himself at his Bellevue farm, and I'm sending the highway patrol to pick you up."

Secretly wishing that Chris had called anyone but me, I hastily cancelled my afternoon patients. Minutes later, a state trooper sped into the front of the Medical Arts Building, and I climbed inside with my black medical bag. With the siren wailing, we headed down Nashville's notorious

Nine Mile Hill toward Bellevue, which, in the 1960s, was still a sparsely populated community of small farmers. When the speedometer reached ninety miles an hour, I asked the trooper to slow down, trying to keep a professional tone to my voice in spite of my anxiety. I was certain that Jesse was already dead, and even if he were alive, there would be little I could do. I had no surgical equipment in my little black bag, and I had no experience treating gun wounds.

My appeal for caution only inspired the trooper to drive faster, so I turned my mind to the task ahead. I had not been close to Chris's grandfather, and I began to look forward to making my first house call in my role as a primary care physician. I hoped to emulate the professional manner of my mentor, Josh Billings, a doctor from the old school. He told famously amusing stories about his house calls, and he had invited me along on many visits to his patients. His liberal use of bourbon as a disinfectant and his reassuring manner had made him a legend among his patients (see Chapter 10).

A short time later, we skidded into Jesse's driveway. I stepped out of the trooper's car and was hit by the sweet smell of cut hay, wet from a recent shower. A few sheep were huddled together in a small pasture, and except for the clucking of chickens in the barnyard, the farm was enveloped in a peaceful silence. It was a misleading prelude to the chaotic and tragic scene inside the farmhouse.

Chris met me in the yard, and I could tell from his face that his grandfather was dead. I felt a wave of sympathy and grief for my cousin. He had been one of my best friends since childhood. We had grown up three blocks from each other and attended the same high school, Montgomery Bell Academy. We both went to Vanderbilt University and although we had taken different professional paths, we remained close friends.

I followed Chris into Jesse's bedroom. He was slumped in his chair with blood covering his shirt and running down his head and neck. Beneath his feet was a pool of fresh blood. Trying to look as professional as possible but feeling afraid and helpless, I began my examination. Jesse was in his nineties and appeared far more frail than I remembered him. He had shot himself once in the chest and once in the head. The weapon, an old revolver that looked like it was left over from the Civil War, was lying at his feet.

I felt grief welling up inside me as I absorbed what Jesse had done. He had managed to shoot himself twice, something I had never heard of. As a meticulous farmer, he had clearly wanted to be certain that he would die. Why had he been so desperate not to survive? What unspoken agony had caused him to take such a decisive and catastrophic action?

Locking It Away

As close as we were, Chris and I never talked about his grandfather's suicide, and whatever questions we had at the time, they remained unasked and unanswered. Today's medical students routinely receive training in grief counseling and end-of-life procedures, but I had no education or experience in handling an unexpected death, much less a suicide.

Looking back, I can see that we were all in a strange kind of denial. I had my own unresolved grief and anger about the death of my father, who was killed by a bolt of lightning on the golf course when I was eighteen. His death and Jesse's suicide remained mysterious and painful to me as a young doctor. I didn't know how to think about them, and I didn't want to. I wanted only to go on living, to be with my family, and take care of my patients. It wasn't until years later that I tried to understand the personal and family consequences of these tragic and violent deaths.

I had no idea what to say or do next. I pronounced Jesse dead. Later I signed off on the coroner's investigation and helped Jesse's daughter make funeral arrangements. It was an era of great reticence about death and dying, and I never spoke with any member of Jesse's family about why he chose suicide as his final solution. Decades later, I learned that he had become too weak to care for himself. A man of deep faith, he was worried about being a burden to his family, and he had chosen to take his own life.

I left the farm with the state trooper, thankful to let Chris take over. On the drive back to Nashville, I was in a subdued and reflective mood. My first house call could not have been more removed from the funny and inspiring stories I had heard from my mentor, Josh Billings. Clearly I had a lot to learn about seeing patients in their homes. If Jesse had been alive, he might have been saved by highly skilled emergency medical care and a quick transfer to the hospital. I was an internist with no training in chest and head wounds, and I would not have known what to do.

At the same time, I felt a strong kinship with physicians in centuries past. They had been called out from their homes day and night. They had picked up their black medical bags and, committed to a mission of healing, they had hurried off to try to help the sick and the dying. The frightened and hope-filled families who met them at the door expected them to save the lives of their loved ones.

I was reminded of a Victorian-era painting by Sir Luke Fildes, entitled *The Doctor*. In the painting, a general practitioner, a GP, is on a home visit to the sick child of a poor laboring family. The doctor is at the bedside, looking with wise intent at the child, while a father stands helplessly in the background, his hand on the shoulder of his tearful wife.*

In reality, the nineteenth-century doctor was nearly as helpless as his patients. He seldom had the training, equipment, or medicines needed to save lives hanging in the balance. His tourniquet was no match for a patient bleeding out from an artery severed by a gunshot wound. He could not give a blood transfusion. He could only watch helplessly while children gasped for breath and then died from diphtheria infections choking off their tiny tracheas. At times, because he had no antibiotics, a doctor could not even save patients from small, infected cuts. Like me at Jesse's death scene, his black bag might as well have been empty.

All the same, the doctor's black bag had been a symbol of a compassionate heart. It was a comforting sign of a doctor willing to visit patients in their homes. As we pulled back into Vanderbilt, I was proud to be in the company of a long line of physicians, doing their best with the limited resources they had at hand.

---

* A physician from that era congratulated Sir Fildes "for showing the world the typical doctor, as we would like to be shown—an honest man and a gentleman, doing his best to relieve suffering. A library of books in our honor would not do what this picture has done and will do for the medical profession in making the hearts of our fellow man warm to us with confidence and affection." *Br J Gen Pract.*, 2008 March 1, 58(548): 210–213

Black Bag

Since my visit to Jesse's farm, I have made hundreds of house calls. Although my mentor, Josh Billings, routinely showed up for home visits with nothing but his wallet, I have always carried my physician's black bag. It reassures patients, and for me, it is also an important symbol of a doctor who cares enough to see patients in their homes.

In my black bag, I carry a blood pressure cuff, instruments for eye and ear exams, and basic supplies and medicines. I also take morphine in prepackaged syringes because it is a must-have narcotic for severe pain.

The "must-have" list varies from doctor to doctor. In medical school, Dr. Thomas Frist taught us to not make house calls without a trocar. The trocar is a hollow, stainless-steel tube with a beveled end that can be inserted into the trachea of a patient with life-threatening breathing problems. The downside is that the insertion requires an incision.

Dr. Frist was a bit of a showman, and his demonstration on how to use a trocar left an indelible impression on me and my fellow students. Secretly, I wondered if he really expected us to perform this invasive procedure outside of a hospital. Fortunately, I never had reason or inclination to use one on a home visit.*

_____

* Tommy Frist was a businessman and doctor, and the father of Bill Frist, Republican Majority Leader of the U.S. Senate from 2003 to 2007.

3

HEAT WAVE

The bald, fifty-two-year-old man lying on the stretcher was critically ill. He weighed two hundred and sixty pounds, his blood pressure was low, and his heart was racing. His skin was cold and wrinkled from an ice bath in the emergency room, and it was covered with red spots after a lifetime of drinking.

It was July 1, 1959, and I was a brand-new resident at Johns Hopkins Hospital in Baltimore, Maryland. I had been assigned to the Osler 6 ward for the night, and Mr. Slapinski was my very first patient. The call had come at 3:00 a.m. from the admitting resident in the emergency room.

"We're sending you a patient who arrived with heatstroke. His temperature is one hundred and eight degrees. He's also vomiting blood, and his blood sugar is two hundred and ninety [a blood sugar reading of one hundred and eighty is cause for concern]. He's been in his upstairs apartment drinking whiskey throughout the heat wave, and I think he has esophageal varices and cirrhosis, too. Good luck."

I would need it. If the admitting resident was right, Mr. Slapinski was a man at death's door with three potentially fatal conditions. He had heatstroke, bleeding veins in his esophagus from scarring of the liver, and a blood sugar level high enough to cause a diabetic coma. His case would challenge the skill of an experienced physician and medical team, but I had been at Hopkins for only three hours. I didn't know the medical staff, and they didn't know me.

As an added complication, Mr. Slapinski was Polish and did not speak English. A neighbor had reported that he lived alone in a low-income apartment without air conditioning, and he drank a pint of alcohol a day. Except for this information, it was impossible to determine Mr. Slapinski's medical history.

"Welcome to Johns Hopkins, Andy," I muttered to myself. "This should be a night to remember."

I had just wrapped up two years as a resident at Vanderbilt. Thanks to Josh Billings, who was then senior professor of medicine at Vanderbilt, I had been offered a third-year residency at The Johns Hopkins Hospital.* It was the opportunity of a lifetime, and Sue and I were elated to be able to take this next step in my medical career. We spent two days in the car driving from Nashville to Baltimore. At my request, Sue quizzed me on the names and doses of the medicines I would be using in the wards. In retrospect, it was a silly exercise—I could easily look up any information I needed—but it calmed my anxiety about heading to an appointment at the country's premier academic medical center.

---

* Josh Billings, with whom I later shared a private practice (see Chapter 10), was the best man in the wedding of A. McGehee Harvey, the renowned chair of the Department of Medicine at Johns Hopkins. Harvey was known to his friends and colleagues as "Mac." Based only on a call from Josh, Mac had accepted me over the phone into this coveted residency program.

Sue and I moved into a small, second-floor apartment just a block from the hospital. Baltimore was in the middle of a heat wave, and it was at least a hundred and one degrees. We were sweating profusely as we unloaded our relatively few possessions.

The next afternoon I went to the hospital to pick up my uniform, assuming that I would start work the following morning. "Congratulations," the attending physician said. "The Osler 6 ward is all yours as of midnight tonight." The Osler 6 ward, which was a premier assignment, had four rooms, each with four critically ill patients separated from one another by curtains. There was also an open ward for twelve patients who were not as ill. In a few hours, I would be in charge of twenty-five patients, not one of whom I had ever examined.*

Shortly before midnight, I arrived at my assignment in a state of high anxiety and excitement. I rounded with the two seasoned residents, Norman Anderson and Charlie Carpenter, and reviewed with them diagnoses and treatment plans for each patient until 2:00 a.m. The names and cases were a dizzying blur.

I had been on my own for just one hour when the emergency room called to say they were sending up Mr. Slapinski. He arrived in a few moments, lying on a gurney and covered with blood. He had vomited into his ice bath in the emergency room, and the water was bright red.

---

* The Osler wards were named for Sir William Osler, one of the most venerated physicians in the history of American medicine. He set up the medical school team structure at Hopkins (attendings, residents, interns, medical students), and this structure was generally adopted by American medical schools.

Like other patients admitted to the Osler 6 ward, Mr. Slapinski did not have a private doctor. He was now a "staff patient" cared for by our medical team of a resident, an intern, two medical students, and nurses. The team was headed by the chief resident, Frank Iber, and the chairman of the medical department, Mac Harvey, neither of whom were typically on the ward at night. As a resident, I was the highest-ranking member of the team, and, despite the fact that the sum total of my experience on the ward was three hours, I was in charge.

Now I understand how Horatio Hornblower felt, I thought to myself. Hornblower was one of my literary heroes. As a junior seaman and a mere acting lieutenant, he was given command of a ship that came under attack in fog.

The first step was to roll Mr. Slapinski on to his hospital bed, a task that took longer than usual because of his morbid obesity. His skin was cold from his ice bath, and his temperature had dropped to a safer one hundred and one degrees. He was still in danger of slipping into shock because of his significant blood loss and the physical hardships of an ice bath. He was also in danger of bleeding to death because heatstroke not only impairs the functioning of the brain, liver, and kidneys, but it also lowers the number of blood platelets needed for normal clotting.

To save Mr. Slapinski, all our interventions had to be done immediately and at once. We needed to give him fluids, insulin, and a blood transfusion, and we needed to find a way to stop the bleeding. Before we could do any of these, we first had to insert an intravenous line into a vein. Unfortunately, Mr. Slapinski's veins were invisible because they were buried in layers of fat.

Today, doctors have the option of inserting an intravenous catheter into the jugular vein in the neck. In the '50s, this was a new and complicated procedure, and none of us on the medical team knew how to do it. My only choice was to do a "cut-down" to the vein, a time-consuming surgical procedure that I had performed just a few times at Vanderbilt.

While I prepared for the cut-down, the intern, Jack Bennett (a recent graduate of Johns Hopkins medical school) tracked down a Sangstaken tube.* This was a large rubber tube, with a pressure gauge, inserted through the nose and into the throat. The lines that held the tube in place were secured to the face mask of a football helmet. Once the tube was in the esophagus, it was inflated, and the pressure on the veins helped stop the bleeding.

I cut through layers of fat and tissue in search of a vein, and talked Jack through the process of getting the football helmet over Mr. Slapinski's large head and securing the lines. It was just the beginning of a long night full of invasive procedures. Mr. Slapinski remained alert and aware of his surroundings the entire time. He never said a word but steadily looked at me with dark, stoic, and questioning eyes. Perhaps he was wondering what other Draconian insults we were contemplating for his poor, massive, and bleeding body.

As I was sewing up the sutures from the cut-down, a nurse tapped me on the shoulder. "Dr. Spickard, the patient in the bed behind you just died."

"What was his diagnosis?"

---

* Jack went on to become a senior investigator in infectious diseases at the National Institutes of Health.

The Ward System:
A Golden Age of Medical Care

My unusual experience with Mr. Slapinski was the beginning of an exhilarating year. I spent most of my waking hours on the medical wards of Johns Hopkins, which represented a "golden age" of medical care for poor and indigent patients.

In that era, like today, the poor, the already sick, and the elderly were often refused insurance by private carriers. One of the few places they could receive outstanding health care was at teaching hospitals. Johns Hopkins was ranked, then and now, as the best teaching hospital in the world. Uninsured patients were admitted to wards of twenty to thirty beds, and they were cared for by a team of residents, interns, medical students, and nurses led by a senior attending physician.

This quality of patient care was impossible to get in another setting. As young physicians, we were on call twenty-four hours a day, seven days a week. If I admitted a patient, I stayed with her until we were finished. If the ward was calm, I could go home for dinner and bed. If something happened while I was gone, the intern was called first, and if he couldn't handle the problem, I was called any time, day or night.

I was learning under fire from some of the best and brightest medical minds in the world, and I couldn't get enough. When I was off the ward, I went to the library or attended medical conferences, trying to soak up the science and art of medicine. It was everything I dreamed a medical education might be.

In the context of contemporary medical training, with its eighty-hour-a-week limitation, this approach seems a bit insane. But for those of us who wanted the experience of taking responsibility for a patient throughout the entire course of his or her illness, it felt like a program to train thoughtful and mature physicians. I believe it created good doctors, with high levels of professionalism and a lifelong commitment to excellence in medical care.

"He was a chronic lunger and has been near death for the past two days." Chronic lungers were terminally ill patients with deteriorating lung function, usually as a result of smoking for years.

I thought of the admonition of my medical school teachers: *Select every day the winning treatments for your patients and prioritize your work.*

"There's no use trying to resuscitate him," I said. "Mr. Slapinski requires all our time and energy, so we'll deal with the body later." After Mr. Slapinski was stable, there would be time enough to pronounce the lung patient dead, meet with his family, and write up the terminal event.

After we finished inserting and inflating the Sangstaken tube, I listened more closely to Mr. Slapinski's lungs. I heard the distinctive sounds of pneumonia. I assumed it was caused by blood that he had aspirated into his lungs, and we added antibiotics to the intravenous line. By then, Mr. Slapinski was wearing a football helmet and receiving intravenous fluids and insulin. He was also getting a blood transfusion and lying under a cooling blanket to bring his body temperature back to normal.

We completed Mr. Slapinski's admission treatment at dawn. The bleeding from his nose and mouth had stopped, and his blood sugar was stable. His temperature was heading down. We had saved him from heatstroke, bleeding esophageal varices, diabetic coma, and pneumonia. Thanks to our heroic medical interventions, he would live to drink another day. Of course, there was a small chance that Mr. Slapinski would stop drinking, take his insulin faithfully, and die in a peaceful old age. Most likely, however, he would die prematurely from the complications of his alcoholism.

There was no family to report to, no one to hear about Mr. Slapinski's incredible story of survival. Physically exhausted but elated, I moved on to my next patient.

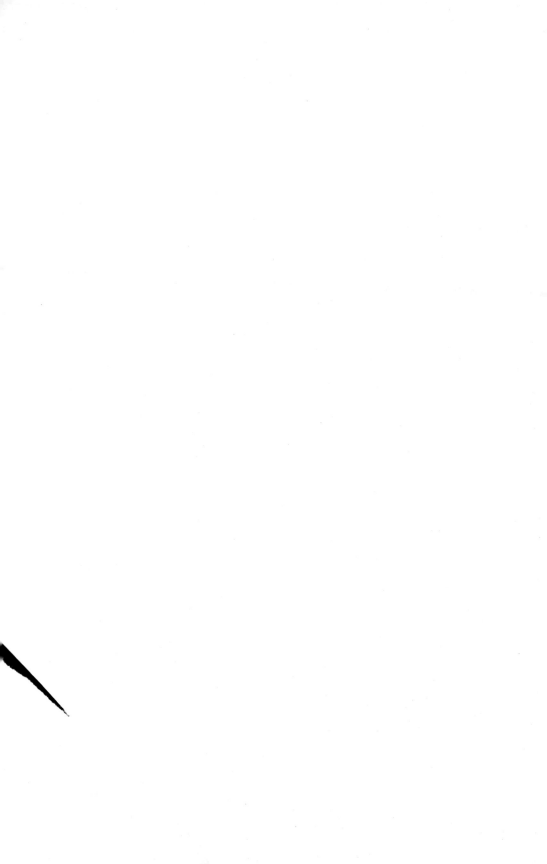

4

TAPEWORM

The diplomat walking casually down the halls of the National Institutes of Health (NIH) looked calmer than he must have felt. He had just returned from a trip to Vietnam, and he had gone to his physician complaining of a minor digestive ailment. The doctor had found evidence of a tapeworm in his stool, and he had appealed to NIH for help. The senior parasitologist at NIH, Dr. Henry Bye, was the world's foremost expert on worms.

It was 1961, and President Kennedy had just moved into the White House. The U.S. involvement in Vietnam had begun. I was a lowly first-year clinical associate at NIH, but it wasn't the first time I had seen a politically connected person admitted to our center. The patients at NIH came from all over the world. Most were suffering from complicated and mysterious illnesses that could not be diagnosed or treated effectively by their primary care doctors. They had fevers of unknown origin, heart infections, and even rare fungal ailments. They were usually admitted to a specific research program for experimental treatments. Occasionally, however, people were accepted because they were politically connected or because, like this diplomat, they played some kind of strategic role in America's foreign policy.

LBJ, I Presume?

One night a colleague of mine was on call to take referrals for new patients. The phone rang, and the caller introduced himself as Lyndon Baines Johnson. The man brusquely explained that he was calling on behalf of a Texas doctor who wanted a patient admitted to NIH to rule out a rare fungus disease.

"If you're Lyndon Baines Johnson," my colleague unwisely responded, "then I am the king of Siam." It *was* Johnson, and while he was not yet the president, he was a powerful, well-connected politician. The patient was admitted and diagnosed with a fungal disease, histoplasmosis, and my hapless colleague received a severe reprimand for his poor telephone protocol.

Dr. Bye asked me and my other first-year colleague, Hugh Evans, to assist him in treating the diplomat. Hugh and I eagerly accepted the invitation. Tapeworm infestation was not common in the United States, and we wanted to see the treatment protocol firsthand. My only other experience with worms had been on the other end of the social scale, with inmates from a federal prison (see Chapter 5). The prisoners were largely poor and from the rural South, and a number had been infected with hookworm from walking barefoot as children or eating dirt.

"This man most likely acquired his tapeworm infection from eating raw pork," Dr. Bye informed us. "Or it might have come from human stool used as fertilizer on rice paddies and vegetable gardens."

He reminded us about what we had learned in medical school textbooks. "The head of the tapeworm, the scolex, attaches to the side of the intestine with very strong teeth. Unless it's expelled forcefully, it can live in the patient for years, causing severe malnutrition."

Hugh and I followed Dr. Bye into the diplomat's room, trying to look like distinguished parasitologists. After talking the patient through the procedure, Dr. Bye inserted a narrow rubber nasogastric tube through his nose and into his stomach. Hugh and I assisted him as he administered Atabrine and magnesium sulfate through the tube. Atabrine was used to force the tapeworm to let go of the intestine wall. Magnesium sulfate softened the patient's stool and helped expel the head of the tapeworm.

"If the medicine doesn't make the head of the tapeworm loosen its grip on the intestine, the treatment will have to be repeated," Dr. Bye explained to the diplomat. The patient appeared to receive this information with professional calm.

When Dr. Bye finished administering the solution, he turned to me and Hugh. "I need you both to be on call around the clock to examine every bit of stool that comes out of the patient. We have to be absolutely certain that the head of the tapeworm has been expelled."

Hugh and I looked at one another. We were by then experienced doctors used to dealing with matters of life and death. Even in our lowly station at NIH as freshmen clinical associates, the task of looking through stool for the head of a tapeworm was an unusual assignment. Unfortunately, saying no to Dr. Bye was not an option.

Hugh and I jokingly referred to the assignment as "stool watch." We set up in a nearby lab for our round-the-clock vigil, taking delivery of the stool as it became available. We conducted rigorous investigations, placing bets on who would be the first to see the scolex.

Fortunately for both of us, the head of the tapeworm appeared less than twenty-four hours later. I do not remember which one of us saw it first. No second treatment or second shift of stool watch was needed. Hugh and I went out to celebrate a messy job well done. For years, we talked over our unusual assignment. "We were freshmen on a sophisticated medical team dealing with high-level political intrigue," I was fond of telling him. "If we could help in some way with the conduct of the war in Vietnam, it was the least we could do."

5

EATON AGENT: AN EXPERIMENT WITH PRISONERS

It should have been a routine case of atypical pneumonia. The patient lying on the hospital bed was a young man with a mildly sore throat and a fever. But his right ear was so inflamed that he could no longer hear out of it, and he was asking for pain medicine.

What made this patient unusual was his prison uniform. He was an inmate volunteer, a willing participant in an experiment designed to increase scientific understanding of the Eaton agent, a microorganism that causes a form of atypical pneumonia.* I had helped make the prisoner sick by giving him an aerosol spray of the infecting agent, and now we had to decide: should the prisoner be removed from the experiment and given an antibiotic?

It was 1962, and I was in my second year as a clinical associate with the Institute for Allergy and Infectious Diseases at the National Institutes

---

* Monroe Davis Eaton was an American bacteriologist who discovered a form of pneumonia seen in humans that was not caused by a bacterium. The pneumonia was described as "atypical" and seemed to resemble viral pneumonia. Atypical pneumonia produces patchy infiltrates in the lungs instead of the consolidated lung infiltrate typical of pneumococcal pneumonia, the more conventional or "lobar" pneumonia. Patients with atypical pneumonia were not as ill and promptly responded to tetracycline, whereas penicillin was usually necessary to treat lobar pneumonia.

of Health. Thanks to President John F. Kennedy, there was growing interest in scientific experiments throughout the country, particularly in the areas of space exploration and medicine. We wanted to do our part at the Institute for Allergy and Infectious Diseases, and much of our research was focused on the causes of respiratory ailments. The Holy Grail of experimental medicine was the cause of the common cold and a vaccine to prevent it.

In this stimulating atmosphere, I was assigned to a team working under the direction of a pediatric researcher, Dr. Bob Channock. Bob had set up an elaborate experiment to prove that a microorganism known as the Eaton agent was a mycoplasma (rather than a virus or a bacterium), *and* that it was the cause of a patchy, atypical pneumonia found in young people in closed environments, like the military or in prisons.

Bob's plan was to follow the rigorous identification and confirmation protocol of Koch's four postulates. Robert Koch, a nineteenth-century medical researcher, was a special hero of mine, and I was happy to participate in an experiment that might identify a disease-causing microorganism and fulfill his postulates.

Our first step was to visit the minimum-security federal prison in Virginia to recruit volunteers and test their level of antibodies to the Eaton agent. The prison was like a dormitory with barred windows and doors, and the prisoners were nonviolent offenders doing time for crimes such as stealing cars and selling bootleg whiskey. As my colleague Hugh Evans and I drew blood from thirty prisoners, the men joked and called out to their friends that they were going to Bethesda to help cure the common cold.

Koch's Postulates

Robert Koch was a German family practitioner. Using the most elementary equipment, he developed dyes and procedures to identify the bacteria that caused tuberculosis. His four famous postulates became the criteria for establishing the causal relationship between a microbe and a disease:

1. The microorganism must be found in abundance in all organisms suffering from the disease, but not in healthy organisms;

2. The microorganism must be isolated from a diseased organism and grown in a pure culture;

3. The cultured microorganism should cause disease when introduced into a healthy organism;

4. The microorganism must be re-isolated from the inoculated, diseased experimental host and identified as being identical to the original specific causative agent.

This human experiment would not be allowed today, but the inmates jumped at the possibility of getting out of prison. In exchange, they received a day off their sentence for every week they spent in the hospital. We were certain that there was minimum risk to the participants, and we knew that they would be closely guarded while at NIH.

The inmate volunteers, dressed in their blue prison uniforms with their numbers on their backs, were brought to NIH by bus. They were assigned two to a room with a guard at the end of each hall. We infected them with the Eaton agent by spraying an aerosol of the infectious organism into their noses and throats. Hugh and I examined the prisoner-patients every day, with a focus on their noses, throats, ears, and lungs. All but seven of the twenty-five with Eaton agent antibodies successfully warded off the infection. Of the twenty-seven without antibodies, twenty became sick with fever, and a physical exam showed inflammation of their lungs.

Three days after the experiment began, a nurse called me to the floor to examine one of the prisoners who was complaining of headache, cough, and an earache. I had wondered how sick the prisoners would get, but I had been assured by reports on military recruits that no one had died from Eaton agent pneumonia. After examining this particular prisoner, however, I was quite concerned. While the other men were mildly ill, he had pneumonia with fever as well as a badly swollen eardrum that made him deaf. He was in so much pain that he was asking for medication. His symptoms shed new light on the potentially serious side effects of Eaton agent pneumonia, and we decided to pull him out of the experiment. We treated him immediately with tetracycline, and his symptoms promptly disappeared.

Meanwhile, we watched colonies of microorganisms growing on the agar plates, and when the colonies were sufficiently large, we took photographs and brought in a specialist to look at them. After pointing out that the technicians had mistakenly photographed the bubbles in the agar, he showed us that right next to the bubbles were the typical fried egg colonies of the Eaton agent. It was clear that the Eaton agent was a mycoplasma rather than a bacterium or a virus.

Bob and our entire team of researchers were elated. The Eaton agent was removed from the agar and put into a new solution, which was sprayed into a second group of prisoners who had tested negative for antibodies to it. These prisoners, too, became ill, and once again, the Eaton agent was grown on agar to identify the cause. Through this elaborate process, we fulfilled all of Koch's postulates and proved that the Eaton agent was the mycoplasma that caused atypical pneumonia.

Throughout the experiment, our relationship with the prisoners was warm and cordial. One inmate, an accomplished artist, drew a picture of my wife holding our firstborn child, Susan, who was newly arrived in the world. This drawing hangs in our home in Nashville to this day.

6

A WOMAN FALLS OUT OF AN ELEVATOR: A QUESTION OF BALANCE

Among the interns and residents at a hospital where I worked one summer in medical school were two young Germans. It had been just ten years since the end of World War II, and they had come to the United States for their residency in hopes of eventually practicing medicine here. In the war, they had been members of the Hitler Youth, a paramilitary organization created by the Nazis. The Germans had drafted twelve-year-olds from the Hitler Youth to create a last line of defense in the Battle of Berlin, and one of the two men boasted that he had manned an anti-aircraft gun to shoot at American planes bombing Berlin.

Oddly, although Germany had taken the world into a war that cost over sixty million lives, I didn't feel animosity toward these young doctors. In all the senseless destruction of World War II, it seemed little short of a miracle that they had survived and made their way to the United States for medical training.

One afternoon, after a meeting with the chief resident, I found myself standing behind the two German residents waiting for an elevator. The elevator door opened, and a woman who was crying and gasping for breath fell out into the hall. She passed out and dropped at their feet.

One of the residents looked at his watch. "It's five o'clock, Spickard," he said. "We're off call. She's your case."

Without a minute's hesitation, both doctors stepped over the unconscious woman and into the elevator. I stood there, open-mouthed. I was an inexperienced medical student with no training in patient care, much less an acute medical emergency. I didn't know how to handle a cardiac resuscitation, and I couldn't even imagine what I was supposed to do next.

A family member knelt over the unconscious woman. "She's just learned that her mother has inoperable cancer and has only a few days to live," she explained, cradling the woman's head in her hands. "I think she's only fainted."

She was right. The woman revived and seemed to recover her equilibrium. I put her feet in the air and checked for vital signs. A chief resident saw me bending over her and stopped to see what was happening. The woman was given fluids in the emergency room and eventually discharged without ongoing problems from falling on the floor.

When she fell, I had been frightened, but after she was sent home, I became angry. I told the chief resident about the doctors' dereliction of duty. They had left an unconscious woman, seemingly in an acute medical crisis, in the hands of a lowly medical student. Had the woman been critically ill, there would have been serious complications for the patient and the hospital. I never knew whether the chief resident reported their behavior, and, fortunately, I never had to work with them again.

A few years later, I was a resident at the Veterans Hospital in Nashville. I walked by a ward supervised by another resident and saw an African American patient struggling to breathe. He clearly needed immediate help, but at that moment, the resident in charge walked out of his room and out the door of the hospital. I learned later that he was on his way to a golf game.

I stared at the doctor's back in disbelief and then went in to see the patient. In between gasps, he said, "Doc, I think I am going to die." The statement itself was an ominous sign. A sense of impending doom is a well-known warning symptom of a heart attack or a pulmonary embolus, which causes instant death.

I called the nurse, who called the attending physician. At that time there was no intensive care at the Veterans Hospital, and the anxious veteran deteriorated rapidly. Within twenty-four hours, he had died of a pulmonary embolus. I never reported the doctor who had abandoned his patient in a true medical emergency. And I never heard what, if anything, he felt about trading responsible patient care for a game of golf.

Balancing Act

The German doctors and the VA resident are two examples, one benign and one fatal, where physicians made the wrong choices in balancing their personal needs with the needs of a patient. Every medical career is full of such choices. Doctors must constantly weigh the needs of their patients with their children's soccer games, family celebrations, or vacations that have been planned for weeks. In medical emergencies, the needs of a patient can exceed a physician's resources. How doctors and their families balance this constant intensity is a critical factor in determining how satisfied doctors are with their medical careers.

(cont.)

Today we teach medical students to care for themselves as well as their patients. Because studies have shown that sleep deprivation can cause critical errors in judgment and performance, residents must limit their work to eighty hours a week. Training programs that don't comply can lose their accreditation.

Medical students today make their choices about future training and practice based on their desire to balance personal and professional life. They are choosing specialties with less need to be on call and to be away from their families at night. This positive trend for medical families has an unfortunate consequence for patients. Specialties like family medicine and primary care internal medicine are not attracting enough doctors because fewer people want to take on the demands of personal patient care. This is particularly so when it comes to the aged and the chronically ill.

To make our family balancing act easier, my wife, Sue, and I made the decision to live close to the hospital. Throughout my career, we never lived more than seven minutes away from my work. I could go back and forth to the hospital and care for patients in unexpected emergencies, while still joining my family for breakfast and dinner (a particularly trying time for young mothers). Whenever I was out of town or on vacation, colleagues who shared my sense of responsibility for patients provided my coverage. It wasn't a perfect system, but it helped create an environment in which both my medical practice and our family could flourish.

7

DEADLY POISON

Monday, October 6, 1963. I was eating lunch in the doctors' dining room at Vanderbilt University with Glenn Koenig, my colleague in the medical school's infectious disease lab. We were talking about a bizarre outbreak of botulism, a rare but potentially fatal disease that had left seven people critically ill in Knoxville. Now there was a rumor that a patient with symptoms of botulism poisoning had shown up at Nashville's General Hospital.

Public health officers in Knoxville had traced the problem to smoked whitefish from Lake Michigan. The fish had been vacuum-packed and improperly stored in a hot warehouse, then distributed by a grocery store chain. The potential for a public health disaster was high, and consumers had been warned about the fish through radio and television announcements. Although I had never seen a patient with botulism, I knew that just one thimble full of the toxin could poison the water supply of an entire town.

Glenn and I were discussing what we would do if the botulism epidemic came to Vanderbilt Medical School, when his beeper went off. It was the emergency room calling. A patient with a history of eating whitefish had just arrived with the symptoms of botulism.

Glenn and I raced to the ER and found a frightened middle-aged man, Raymond, who was struggling to breathe. He had heard about the botulism outbreak on the radio, and he came to the emergency room with a package of whitefish in his hands.

"I can't swallow and my vision is blurry," Raymond said weakly. He had been vomiting, and we could see that his mouth and tongue were extremely dry. One eye was totally sightless due to a previous injury, but the pupil of his good eye was dilated and not reacting to light. The muscles in his face and neck were beginning to freeze, and his breathing was labored. All the symptoms pointed to the descending paralysis that is the hallmark of botulism poisoning.

Botulism: Classic Symptoms

- dilated, nonreactive pupils

- severe dryness of the mouth and tongue

- respiratory muscle paralysis

- varying degrees of abdominal distension

- weakness of muscles in face, neck, arms, and legs

- swelling of the throat

- low blood pressure

- patient remaining mentally alert and clear

We knew we had to act quickly if we were going to save Raymond's life. We performed an emergency tracheotomy to maintain his airway and placed him in an iron lung. It was the same kind of iron lung that I had used in 1956 as a third-year medical student caring for polio victims—modern mechanical ventilators did not come into widespread use until later.

The antidote for fish-related botulism was only available in Denmark, and we had to wait two days for it to arrive.* By then, five other victims of botulism poisoning had died of cardiac arrest and respiratory failure. Among the dead were a father and young daughter from Knoxville.

I was Raymond's chief caretaker throughout his slow recovery. The botulism continued to compromise his breathing, and he was forced to stay in the iron lung. While there, he had a heart attack and developed a urinary tract infection that turned into blood poisoning. Fortunately for the sake of his much-needed lab work, I had learned from polio patients to draw blood through the machine ports of an iron lung by carefully timing the patient's respirations.

Raymond's only family member was his elderly mother, and he had no visitors.† I spent so much time with him during his long ordeal that we became friends. He kept his sense of humor and optimism, and I looked forward to our daily visits. After two weeks, he was released from the iron lung with no disabling complications. He returned home to continue caring for his mother and direct his neighborhood bowling league.

---

* The Type E botulism in infected fish was not the same botulism (Type A and Type B) found in canned food. Because botulism poisoning from canned food was much more common, the antidote was also more readily available.
† Raymond's elderly mother had eaten the same meal of whitefish but did not become ill. We learned that she had used an enema the night after eating the whitefish. Because it took twelve hours for the bacteria to produce symptoms of botulism, we speculated that she had expelled it from her colon.

Missed Diagnosis

In the aftermath of the botulism epidemic, I participated in an epidemiological study with Glenn Koenig and David Rogers, then chairman of medicine at Vanderbilt. As a relatively new doctor, it was my first experience diagnosing a rare disease, providing direct patient care, and conducting research with a team of brilliant and like-minded doctors.

We identified eight patients from Nashville and Alabama who had symptoms of botulism poisoning, and we injected white mice with their blood. The test confirmed that all eight had Type E botulism.

We then reviewed the patients' clinical histories and the quality of their care. Although the outbreak of botulism was widely known in the medical community, and all eight patients exhibited its classic symptoms, seven patients were misdiagnosed. Of these seven, three died. Their physicians no doubt believed that their patients had died from a heart attack or stroke. The rate of misdiagnosis illustrated the rarity of botulism poisoning and underscored how difficult it is for doctors to diagnose an uncommon and unexpected disease.

8

TO AN ATHLETE
(ALMOST) DYING YOUNG

It was September 1 at a small liberal arts college in the middle of Tennessee, and the football team was practicing twice a day. Jim, an aspiring running back, was exhausted. He had lost six pounds in the morning practice and was too hot and tired to eat lunch. In the afternoon, he dressed in full uniform for two-on-one blocking drills, tackling, and running dummy offensive plays. Then he began running up a thirty-yard hill with his teammates. After two runs, he did not know where he was. On the eighth run, he collapsed. A fellow player rushed to his side, took one look at Jim's face, and called out, "Coach, Jim is dying!"

The head coach rushed over to Jim. "His eyes were sunken, and his pupils were getting bigger," he later reported. "He was completely motionless and was barely breathing."

Like the other players, Jim had received a precursory physical the day before practice, and he had been declared fit to play. The exam for high school and college athletes, which hasn't changed much over the years, focused on heart and lung function, and checked for a hernia and the testicular cancer mass that is found in some young males.

Nothing in the exam would have predicted what was happening to Jim. But as a big running back, his extreme weight loss in the morning practice was a critical warning sign that might have been caught by his coaches. Jim was now having heatstroke—hyperthermia—and his body could not control its own skyrocketing temperature. He was in imminent danger of death, and even if he survived, he was likely to have significant kidney and liver damage.

With his coaches and fellow players looking on with fear, Jim was loaded into an ambulance and rushed to the local hospital. A body temperature of one hundred and four degrees is considered a critical emergency in a heatstroke patient. Jim arrived at the ER with a body temperature of one hundred and eight, ten degrees above normal. He was immediately put in a cool bath and given oxygen and saline solution, as well as Dilantin and Valium to control his spasmodic seizures and skyrocketing blood pressure.

Jim's blood tests showed severe damage to his kidneys and liver, caused by the exposure of his body tissues to intense heat over a prolonged period of time. His high body heat was literally singeing his vital organs, including his brain and heart. He was already suffering from reduced urine output from kidney failure, and he was turning yellow from jaundice of the liver.

When Jim was relatively stabilized, his doctor called me to see if we could take him at the Vanderbilt Hospital. The doctor was afraid that Jim was going to die. If he lived, he knew that Jim would require long-term hospitalization to manage the fluids and nutrition that his body needed to repair the damaged tissue of his vital organs. If Jim's kidneys permanently failed, he would also need lifelong renal dialysis.

When Jim arrived at Vanderbilt, one look at his face told me that he was in serious trouble. I thought of the six soldiers who had died the previous summer of heatstroke during basic training at Fort Campbell on the Kentucky-Tennessee border. I had been consulting on infectious diseases for the 101st Airborne Infantry, and I had not been able to forget the sad photo of their young bodies laid out on a tarpaulin.

Jim was far luckier, probably because he received treatment more quickly. After three weeks of critical care in our intensive care unit, he completely recovered from his heatstroke, without long-term complications to any of his vital organs. We explained to Jim that once a person has suffered heatstroke, he is at high risk for a reoccurrence. Jim wisely chose not to play football again, but he returned to college and graduated with his class.

· · · · ·

Some time later, I saw another young football player with heatstroke. Phil was a tackle who had become sick while practicing during an unexpected heat wave in November. He was sent to the locker room. Fortunately his father was watching practice from the stands. He thought his son had only gone to the bathroom, and when Phil didn't return, he went to find him in the locker room.

He found Phil fallen on the floor, disoriented and on the edge of consciousness. He didn't know his son was having a life-threatening heatstroke, but he had the presence of mind to immediately call an ambulance. Because of his quick action, we were able to save his son's life at Vanderbilt Hospital. Phil eventually graduated from Vanderbilt Law School.

I knew from research done in Israel that Phil had probably lost his acclimatization to heat. By studying young soldiers in the desert, the Israelis had learned that soldiers gradually exposed to increases in temperature

41

could adapt to the demands of strenuous exercise. Their adrenal glands protected their vital organs by lowering the loss of sodium through sweat and urine. Without acclimatization, the brain's heat control mechanism could collapse and lead to death.

With Jim's and Phil's near-death experiences on my mind, I went to the Vanderbilt machine shop and asked them to create a heat thermometer similar to one at Fort Campbell. This tri-part thermometer was used for years by the Vanderbilt football team during the hot days of summer practice and whenever there was a late-season heat wave.

We published two papers from Vanderbilt on heatstroke, and the conclusions drawn from this research have been widely disseminated to high school, college, and pro football coaches.* There are clear and well-known guidelines for exercising in hot weather. Nonetheless, from 1995 to 2009, twenty-nine young football players have died from heatstroke. The deaths of these talented, hard-working young people are all the more tragic because the deaths were, and are, completely preventable.

---

* Spickard A, "Heatstroke in College Football and Suggestions for Prevention," *So Med J*, 61: 791–796, 1968; Spickard A, Worden J, "How to Prevent Heatstroke in Football Players," *J Nat Athletic Trainers Assoc* 3: 6–9, 1968

A Life-Saving Thermometer

After the tragic, unnecessary deaths of six soldiers from the 101st Airborne, the U.S. Armed Forces created a comprehensive program to prevent heatstroke in trainees. The prevention strategy included determining the heat index, which was calculated from the measurements of three thermometers: a wet and a dry bulb, and a black globe thermometer.

At Fort Campbell, the thermometers were positioned on an outdoor stand, and senior officers calculated the heat index as measured by the three thermometers. When the temperature reached a dangerous level, the officers sounded a siren and training ended immediately. Any officer who continued training was subject to court martial. This strategy is now the required procedure for all military personnel at training sites.

9

THE COZY HORSEHAIR CHAIR

I found Joe slumped over in his horsehair chair, holding a glass full of vodka. The ice cooler at his elbow held two large bottles, strategically placed so that he never needed to get up to refill his glass. A black-and-white television was running in the background.

Joe's wife had called me earlier in the day, begging me to make a house call on her semicomatose husband. "He needs help, but he won't leave his chair," she explained. "Someone has to do something!"

Joe was not only my patient but a boyhood friend. We had gone to the same school as teenagers, and we played football together in a field across from his family's home. As a boy, I never dreamed that I would one day return to that same house as a medical doctor, wondering what I could possibly do to save my old friend from drinking himself to death.

The man I saw sitting in the horsehair chair was nothing like the fun-loving and talented athlete I had known as a boy. Instead, he was a living monument to all the ways alcohol could destroy a human body. His nose was swollen, his face red and blotchy, and his eyes were yellow from the bile his liver was no longer able to process. His stomach was bloated from cirrhosis, the scarring of his liver.

I knew that Joe was a "sippin'" alcoholic. He drank enough alcohol around the clock to keep himself intoxicated but never enough to get into fights or fall over. He wasn't in danger of getting a DWI because he never left his home. In fact, he didn't even need to get up. His wife and kids kept his cooler stocked, and he was free to spend his days and nights in his horsehair chair, sipping.

To examine Joe, I needed to get him out of his chair, which had formed a kind of body cast around him. It was not an easy task, but with the help of his wife and daughter, I got him onto a bed. Within minutes, I knew that Joe was in the final stages of alcoholism. His liver was enlarged and barely functioning, and his lack of normal reflexes suggested severe damage to the nerves in his legs and feet. He could not remember a simple series of three items, and he was even having trouble recalling his wife's name.

At the time, I had very little education in the treatment of alcoholism, but I knew enough to know that Joe was about to die in his horsehair chair. I called an ambulance and sent him straight to Vanderbilt for detoxification. We administered nutrients and vitamins to try to prevent further brain damage, but it was too late. Joe was already suffering from Wernike-Korsakoff syndrome, an end-stage dementia caused by chronic alcoholism. (This syndrome might have been prevented by a vitamin regime including thiamine or even simply a modestly healthy diet.) Despite our best medical efforts to control his disorientation, he was confused by his hospitalization. He mistook his wastebasket for a urinal and tried to climb out the window of a seven-story tower. His brain was far too damaged to ever recover. Because there was nothing more to be done, the hospital sent him home.

I made one more house call at the request of Joe's wife. Joe was still sitting in the horsehair chair, sipping vodka. His liver was almost in complete failure, and his severe jaundice was causing fluid retention, with both his legs and stomach swollen to three times their normal size. His heart rhythm was erratic, and he was experiencing not only dropped beats but rapid runs. It was a sign that the muscles of the heart were wearing out, along with the delicate mechanism that controlled his heartbeat and pulse.

This time I sent Joe to a nursing home. He died there a few weeks later when he fell and hit his head on the bathtub. To this day, I can still see that horsehair chair and the deep imprint that Joe's body had made on it. It remains a haunting image for me of my boyhood friend, and the comfortable, cozy way his promising life was drowned by alcohol.

10

DEAD MAN BREATHING

I was introduced to the art of making house calls by a master of the trade, Josh Billings. Josh was a legend even among his highly accomplished peers, and he was the most influential colleague, teacher, and friend in my medical life. He taught me that a good doctor makes a point to learn more about his or her patients than the simple facts of their disease.

Josh believed that house calls enabled him to understand his patients in the broader context of their lives. They also allowed him to observe the role that home environment might play in an illness. His patients and their families were overwhelmed with gratitude when he made a home visit. Their experience of his deep personal concern seemed as important, or more important, than any medicine he gave them.

Josh loved to tell the story of one of his most unusual house calls. One night, the wife of a sixty-five-year-old patient telephoned him to say that her husband had died at home. Would Josh come pronounce him dead? Josh advised the woman to call an ambulance, but she insisted that he come to the scene himself. This was in the days before a coroner was required to rule out the possibility of foul play.

Josh went to the couple's upstairs apartment and pronounced the husband dead. He appeared to have died from a heart attack. "Would you take him over to Vanderbilt?" the wife asked. "He wanted his body to be donated to the anatomy department."

In the spirit of "in for a penny, in for a dollar," Josh agreed. Finding bodies for anatomy classes was not an easy task, and like all of us in the medical school, Josh was committed to helping students get the corpses they needed.

It was 2:00 a.m. when Josh loaded the dead man's body on his back in a fireman's carry and started down the stairs. With each jarring step, the man's body took a bounce. Eventually the pressure on his abdomen caused air to escape from his lungs and mouth. The wife, who was trailing behind Josh, heard the rush of air and thought her husband was breathing.

Josh Billings had an exclusive group of rich and famous patients from the prestigious Belle Meade neighborhood of Nashville. He made home visits there and could charm even the most demanding and irritating patients.

Late one afternoon, a wealthy patient asked him if he could come by her house on his way home to look at her exceptionally painful sore throat. Josh agreed. Because he never traveled with a medical bag or carried medical supplies, he stopped at a pharmacy to buy a syringe, some penicillin, a tongue blade, and a roll of cotton. He put the supplies in his pocket, and when the butler answered the door, he asked for a flashlight so that he could examine his patient's throat. He also asked for some bourbon. He poured the bourbon in a glass, and used it to soak his cotton ball and wipe off the syringe and the patient's arm. Then he gave her a shot of penicillin.

When the woman recovered, she told all her friends about Josh and his liberal use of bourbon. This story raised Josh's standing even higher, and he never lacked for new and well-to-do patients.

"He's alive! Dr. Billings, my husband is alive!"

Staggering under the weight of the body, Josh tried to assure the woman that her husband really was dead. She continued to scream. The weight of the body was too much for Josh, and at the bottom of the stairs, he dropped the deceased man on a Turkish rug. He explained to the shocked wife why her husband's body appeared to be breathing, and then he used the rug to pull the body out to the curb. By then, there was more than one neighbor watching from the apartment windows.

Josh's car was an old Checker Cab that he had driven for years. He shouldered the dead man into the back seat, and for the benefit of neighbors and passing cars, he propped up the body to make it look like it was only a man sleeping. He sped to the emergency room at Vanderbilt, praying that he would not be stopped by a policeman. He stayed around long enough to make sure the corpse was transferred to the anatomy department and then went home to bed.

For Josh Billings, the master of the house call, it was all in a night's work.

Scholar, Athlete, War Hero, Friend

F. Tremaine "Josh" Billings Jr., MD

1912–2007

Josh Billings was the ultimate example of what a good doctor should be: honest and careful.

As a student, Josh attended Choate and then Princeton, where he captained the football team and won the Pyne Prize, the school's highest honor. He was a Rhodes Scholar and contracted polio while studying at Oxford University. After his recovery, he went to Johns Hopkins for medical school and did postdoctoral medical training at both Johns Hopkins and Vanderbilt.

During World War II, a month after he was married in 1942, Josh joined the Hopkins medical unit in the Pacific theater. He was later discharged as a lieutenant colonel, and, after the war, he practiced internal medicine in Nashville. He was a professor of medicine at Vanderbilt University Medical Center and served as dean of the medical students. He helped create a partnership between Vanderbilt and Meharry Medical School, a historically black school in Nashville, where he became chair of the department of medicine. Josh also pioneered a health program for rural Appalachia.

Josh was my teacher in my third year of medical school, and after my training in infectious diseases at Johns Hopkins and NIH, he invited me into his private medical practice in Nashville. The five years we worked together were some of the most personally and professionally rewarding of my medical career.

When I was on call for Josh, he left instructions about which patients should be visited at home. Likewise, when his patients came to the emergency room without first notifying him, the staff knew to call Josh immediately, day or night. As a primary care physician, he knew far more than any other doctor about his patients' illnesses, and he insisted on signing off on every diagnosis and treatment plan.

In 2000, Princeton University chose Josh Billings to be its "Scholar-Athlete of the Century." As a man and a physician, Josh Billings left such a profound impression on Sue and me that we named our second son David Billings Spickard.

11

THE GREAT TREE EPIDEMIC

"Hey, Doc, I can't breathe. Please do something!"

Mark was lying on a bed in the intensive care unit in Williamson County, Tennessee, and turning blue from lack of oxygen. He had a fever and chronic cough, and his X-ray showed numerous small patches of infection throughout his lungs. His wheezing and decreased breath sounds suggested a widespread infection of pneumonia, but his blood tests didn't support the diagnosis. He had already been given broad-spectrum antibiotics and nasal oxygen, but these remedies were not working.

I was an infectious disease specialist as well as an associate professor of internal medicine at Vanderbilt Medical Center. Because Mark's symptoms were so puzzling, his primary care doctor, Dr. Bob Hollister, had called me in for a consult. He suspected that Mark had been infected by the *Histoplasma capsulatum* fungus found in bird and bat droppings. If so, he needed to know how to treat this relatively rare lung condition.

I learned that twelve days earlier, on Mother's Day, Mark had thrown a party for his friends and neighbors. The previous night, a violent thunderstorm had struck Williamson County and toppled an ancient and partially rotten white oak tree in front of Mark's house. It was the largest tree in the area and had been a neighborhood landmark. Mark invited forty-two friends to help him cut up and clear the tree. The guests brought rakes and saws, and axes and chainsaws. With their wives and families, they settled in for a grand weekend event of eating and drinking and socializing. Five dogs were also present.

Some of the partygoers reported that they had seen a large cloud of dust coming out of the tree as they cut it up with chainsaws. I suspected that the cloud carried the remains of starling nests that were loaded with histoplasma fungus. Mark had likely breathed the spores deeply into his lungs. As his white cells attacked the invading organisms, his air sacs became inflamed and incapable of transferring oxygen to the blood. Now without appropriate treatment, Mark's breathing would become even more severely compromised, and his illness would likely end in death. Ironically, he had with him a photograph of himself sitting victoriously on the fallen oak, blissfully unaware that the fungus-laden tree was infecting him with a life-threatening illness.

Mark was put in a critical care unit, and his physical condition deteriorated rapidly. Meanwhile, more people from his tree-cutting party were coming into the emergency room with symptoms of coughing and low-grade fever. None had the level of infection from which Mark was suffering, but they had heard about his condition and were worried that they might have the same illness.

I advised Dr. Hollister to begin treating Mark with Amphotericin-B, the fungal antibiotic specific for histoplasma infection. I also called the Centers for Disease Control (CDC) in Atlanta. I explained that there was a growing group of people with similar symptoms of infection from a common source, and they immediately sent an infectious disease officer to the county to do a detailed survey and assessment.

54

The laboratory work of the CDC confirmed that the area was in the midst of a "Great Tree" epidemic. Although Mark had the most extended exposure and was understandably the sickest, three-quarters of the participants in the tree party had been infected with the histoplasma fungus. Almost half had pulmonary disease, and three required hospitalization. Two of the five dogs also developed serious lung disease.

Histoplasmosis: Childhood Legacy

My colleagues and I wrote up the story of the "Great Tree Epidemic" in the *American Journal of Medicine,* and it became a seminal paper on histoplasma infection.* Other smaller epidemics of histoplasmosis disease connected to starlings roosting in trees and shrubs have been reported in medical journals. Medical students learn that farmers can get histoplasmosis by cleaning out a chicken house.

Ironically, I have the scars of histoplasma infection in my eye. The likely cause is a childhood chore. My family raised chickens in our backyard in Nashville, and my job was to clean the roosts. My scars, which do not affect my vision, have been a source of endless curiosity for generations of Vanderbilt ophthalmology residents. Their understanding of fungus infections is enriched every time I have an eye exam.

* Ward JI, Weeks M, Allen D, Hutcherson R Jr., Anderson R, Fraser DW, Kaufman L, Ajello L, Spickard A, "Acute Histoplasmosis: Clinical Epidemiologic and Serologic Findings of an Outbreak Associated with Exposure to a Fallen Tree," *Amer J of Med*, 66, 587–595, 1979

Mark and the rest of the infected patients, including the dogs, responded well to treatment. They all recovered completely. As the sickest patient, Mark was short of breath for a few weeks, but gradually his breathing returned to normal. Like many people exposed to histoplasma spores, he had buckshot-sized calcifications in his lungs for the rest of his life. These scars did not compromise his breathing, but they remained visible proof of a party that he wished he had never hosted.

12

TYPHOID MARY

My first encounter with Mary, a domestic worker in Nashville, was for a routine checkup. She was applying for a job as a family maid, and the state required all food handlers and domestic workers to get a skin test for tuberculosis and a blood test for syphilis. Both tests for Mary came back negative, and I signed her health card saying she was free from transmissible disease. Mary went off to work in a suburban Nashville home, and I did not expect to hear from her again.

Six months later, I received a call from a Nashville pediatrician who had been my roommate in medical school. He wanted me to examine a four-year-old child who had tested positive for typhoid fever, a rare disease in the United States. Although millions of people came down with typhoid every year in countries with poor public sanitation and impure water, there were only four hundred or so victims annually in the United States. Most of these people had returned from overseas travel, and a few had consumed food or drink handled by an infected restaurant worker.

By the time I examined the child, whose name was Daniel, he was well on his way to recovery. He was no longer running a high fever or having diarrhea, and his skin rash, the bright rose-colored spots of typhoid, was disappearing. He was on ampicillin, the preferred antibiotic for typhoid fever, and he was eating well. His only problem was that he wanted to go home.

Still, a mystery remained. How could a little boy who had never traveled out of the United States come down with typhoid fever in Nashville? Since the public water supply was not a suspect, the most likely possibility was that Daniel had crossed paths with a typhoid carrier, a person who had recovered from typhoid but was still acting as a host for the typhoid bacillus. The contagion was generally not a question of personal hygiene: it is virtually impossible for typhoid carriers to wash their hands thoroughly enough to kill the typhoid bacteria.

The most famous carrier in the United States had been "Typhoid Mary." The New York City cook and domestic worker had caused fifty-three cases of typhoid and three deaths during her bizarre and extended career as an infectious agent. She refused to quit working and would have infected many more people had she not been arrested by health authorities in New York City. Mary was placed in permanent quarantine on an island until her death twenty-three years later in 1938.

To find the source of Daniel's typhoid, we tested his entire family and their maid, who turned out to be Mary, the woman to whom I had given a clean bill of health just six months earlier. We also tested the water in the creek that ran in front of the family's home, where Daniel and his friends routinely played. The water and the stool samples from the family members came back negative. All three of Mary's stool samples tested positive for typhoid bacillus.

As Mary's doctor, it fell to me to break the bad news to her and arrange for the appropriate medical interventions. It was an unpleasant but necessary task. Like her famous namesake, Mary was adamant that she could not be a carrier for typhoid. She did not remember ever having an illness like Daniel's, and her digestion had always been good.

Reluctantly, Mary agreed to come back to the Vanderbilt Clinic for a complete exam. An ultrasound of her gallbladder showed one of the largest stones I had ever seen. This stone was almost certainly the origin of Daniel's typhoid infection. At some point in Mary's life, she had been exposed to typhoid bacillus, and the stone had formed around the infection. The porous walls of the stone enabled the infection to travel with the bile through her liver and down to the bowel, where it became a permanent source of infection in her stool.

Mary remained adamant that she could not be a typhoid carrier, and it was difficult to convince her to have the stone taken out. Finally, she agreed. The surgeon removed a stone, four by two inches, and then gave it to me for laboratory analysis. I washed its exterior carefully with a solution designed to kill all the typhoid germs on its surface. Then I placed the stone in a flask of broth that would grow typhoid organisms. Within twenty-four hours, the culture was teeming with typhoid organisms, proving that Mary's gallbladder was the source of Daniel's typhoid.

In a time before antibiotics, the original Typhoid Mary had to be forcibly quarantined. Nashville's Typhoid Mary was more fortunate. The remaining typhoid organisms in her body were killed by ampicillin, and she received a clean certificate for work as a domestic worker.

Like her namesake, Mary continued to adamantly deny that she was the source of the infection. Although I assured her repeatedly that it was not a case of personal responsibility—she could not have known about her infection, and it would have been impossible to kill the typhoid bacillus every time she washed her hands—I suspect she felt guilty nonetheless. She never came back to see me in the clinic again.

13

A MERCIFUL DEATH

Sherrie sat across from my desk, holding a red-tinged tissue to the side of her mouth. Her face was shockingly disfigured from a chronic infection called lethal midline granuloma. Her nose and mouth were partly eroded, and she could barely swallow because the infection had traveled to her tongue and the roof of her mouth. She needed the tissue to absorb the constant bloody drool that dripped from her lips.

It was 1968. I was thirty-seven, and I was in private practice in Nashville with Josh Billings. Sherrie's disease was in an advanced stage, and I suspected that she had come to me as a last desperate effort to get another opinion and another course of treatment. My heart broke as I looked at this beautiful woman and reviewed what I knew of her case. The cause of lethal midline granuloma was unknown, and as far as I knew, there was no successful course of treatment. Radiation, steroids, and cancer medications sometimes slowed down the progression of the disease, but patients usually had less than two years to live. Most often they died from bleeding.

I told Sherrie that I would research her illness in the medical literature and find out if there were treatments that I didn't know about. Meanwhile, I admitted her to Vanderbilt Hospital, so that consultants could take biopsies and cultures in search of an intervention that might help prolong her life.

In the end, there was nothing we could do. The medications were useless, and radiation only made her fragile tissues bleed more profusely. After only a week, we had to send Sherrie home to await an inevitable death from pneumonia or bleeding. I felt enormous respect for her as I witnessed the bravery and stoicism with which she accepted her prognosis. She had already endured overwhelming pain and fear, and her courage moved me even more deeply than her tears.

Shortly after Sherrie was discharged from the hospital, her daughter called me frantically to say that her mother was bleeding uncontrollably. Would I come to the house? I called an ambulance to meet me at their home, and then I raced out the door, knowing that I might arrive too late to be of any help.

I found Sherrie hemorrhaging profusely from a hole at the top of her mouth, where she had a large erosion. There was nothing I could do to stop her bleeding. Only surgical intervention could save her life now. When the ambulance arrived, we all worked quickly with her daughter to get Sherrie onto a gurney. Within minutes, she was on her way to the hospital, which was twenty minutes away.

I rode in the ambulance with Sherrie, holding her as she bled uncontrollably. I felt sick that there was nothing I had been able to do to prevent the impending death of this precious woman. I also felt afraid because I was pretty certain that we were not going to make it to the hospital in time. I had patients die under my care as a resident, but this was totally different. I was Sherrie's primary physician, and if she bled to death in my arms, I would be with her during her last moments on earth. How would I know what to do?

I had never discussed Sherrie's faith journey with her, and I had no idea if she had a pastor or priest who might have been helpful to her. Later in my career, I made a point of asking patients about their spiritual beliefs, but all I knew about Sherrie was the deep respect, sympathy, and love that I felt for her.

I found myself praying for her and for myself, that I could be for this extraordinary woman whatever she needed. It came to me that she had suffered enough and that the end of her life would be the beginning of her healing. All I could do, and all I needed to do, was to stay with her, to hold her while she made her passage to eternal life.

Sherrie died quietly in my arms in the ambulance. In the end, it was a painless and merciful death.

14

THE KILLER AIR CONDITIONER

The mid-afternoon sun was beginning to cast shadows through my office window as I sat down to talk with my ninth patient of the day. Elizabeth was an attractive young lawyer in her middle twenties, dressed in an expensive brown suit and coat. The poise and professionalism with which she had entered my office had evaporated. She was wringing her hands with anxiety and squinting, as if she had forgotten to wear her glasses.

"A friend of mine was just recently diagnosed with a brain tumor," she said, with fear in her voice. "Now I have some of her same symptoms."

For a moment, I wondered if Elizabeth was overidentifying with her friend. But as she began explaining her symptoms, she quickly had my full attention. There was a pain in the back of her neck, which was worse when she bent over. She had not suffered an injury. She was experiencing a severe headache on both sides of her forehead, and her vision had been blurred for almost two weeks.

It was the kind of case that sometimes makes medicine not only tantalizing but filled with a sense of foreboding. I had seen a thousand patients with garden-variety headaches, but Elizabeth's symptoms were not routine. Unlike stress-related headaches, her pain was increasing in intensity. Combined with the pain in her neck, her blurred vision, and the absence of any injury, it suggested that pressure was building up in her brain and on the nerves in her skull.

I mentally created an algorithm of her symptoms and the causes of intracranial pressure. I could rule out bacterial meningitis because of its acute onset and associated fever. It might be inflammation of the blood vessels in the brain, but this was most common in older people. Besides, Elizabeth did not have the muscle aches associated with the disease.

There was really only a handful of possibilities, and all of them were serious: a brain tumor, a hemorrhage, or an infection caused by tuberculosis or a fungus. My physical exam of Elizabeth helped narrow the possibilities. Her blood pressure, pulse, and temperature were normal, but when I asked her to bend her head forward, she let out a scream. Her acute pain suggested a brain hemorrhage and the accumulation of blood around the spinal cord, or chronic meningitis. Chronic meningitis is a life-threatening infection of the central nervous system caused by tuberculosis or a fungus.

Like most cases, it was a process of elimination. At the time, I did not have computerized tomography to rule out a brain tumor, but I knew that a tumor would not cause pain when she bent her head. If Elizabeth was having a brain hemorrhage, most likely her symptoms would have come on more quickly. That left only fungus or tuberculous meningitis as the likely cause of her symptoms.

When I examined Elizabeth's optic nerves, I saw that both optic discs were swollen. This swelling accounted for her blurred vision, and it added evidence for a diagnosis of meningitis (an infection of the meninges, the three-layer membrane covering the brain and spinal cord). She would need a spinal tap to sort out whether this infection was caused by tuberculosis or fungus disease.

After Elizabeth underwent a painful spinal tap, I looked at her spinal fluid under a microscope. In the India ink preparation, I could easily see that she had acquired cryptococcal meningitis, an infection caused by inhaling the dust of bird droppings. The organisms had first lodged themselves in her lung tissue, and then her blood had carried them to her brain and spinal cord. There they were causing a life-threatening inflammation of the meninges.

Fortunately for Elizabeth, the cryptococcus organism was highly sensitive to an antifungal agent, Amphotericin-B. She was given this drug intravenously every day for six weeks, and we did periodic spinal taps to assess her progress and relieve the pressure in her head and neck. Elizabeth responded quickly, and she recovered without the complication of reoccurring infection that occurs in some people with meningitis.*

· · · · ·

In Elizabeth's case, however, a problem still remained. We did not know how she had become infected. Until we knew the answer, it was possible, perhaps even likely, that she could become sick again. I asked Elizabeth if she had been exposed to any bird droppings. "Yes," she said emphatically. "I've been worried about some starlings that are making nests in our attic. And I've heard them around the air conditioner."

From my studies at the National Institutes of Health, I knew that, in the 1950s, a researcher by the name of Chester Emmons had investigated the high incidence of cryptococcal meningitis occurring in government employees in Washington, DC. Emmons found that pigeons and other birds perched on the ledges of government buildings were producing droppings infected with cryptococcus. Dust from these droppings created a dangerous aerosol, and office workers were becoming sick simply by breathing.

---

* Patients with impaired immunity from an underlying disease, such as Hodgkin's lymphoma or AIDS, are at risk for relapse. They have trouble fighting off the cryptococcal infection, and residual organisms remaining in the spinal fluid may reappear once the drug regimen ends.

I asked Elizabeth if I could investigate her home, and she agreed. It was the first and only time I made a house call on an air conditioner. It turned out to be a critical step in Elizabeth's recovery. I found the attic full of bird excreta and dust. The air conditioner, which stood just below the broken attic vent, was also covered with bird droppings. Inside was a dead starling that had come in through a hole in the casing.

In the kitchen, I saw that the air conditioner blew right across Elizabeth's seat at the table. When she was eating during hot weather, it was likely that she was also breathing a steady stream of infected dust into her nose, throat, trachea, and lungs. To confirm my suspicion, I removed the air conditioner from the window and brought it back to the laboratory at Vanderbilt. I made multiple cultures of the dust and starling droppings, looking for the cryptococcus organisms.

Because I wasn't an expert on the process of culturing, I never was able to confirm beyond any doubt that the air conditioner was the source of Elizabeth's infection. At the same time, I remembered the words of one of my favorite detectives on the television series *Hawaii Five-0*. "You've been trained to recognize the unusual," he told a colleague. "So when the facts in a case don't add up, trust your instincts." My instincts told me that the air conditioner was the source of the problem.

Even without absolute proof, the public health authorities closed Elizabeth's house until every room, including the attic, could be cleaned and fumigated. When Elizabeth had recovered enough to return home, she did so reluctantly. She and her husband decided to sell their house, but it remained on the market for a long time. No one wanted to buy the house with the killer air conditioner.

15

TAKE YOUR SECRET TO THE GRAVE

"Don't say a word to anyone."

Andrew was the head of his department in a midwestern medical school, and he had been found in bed with one of his patients. The patient's husband was threatening to sue Andrew and the school, and go to the newspapers. The dean of the medical school called me because he knew that Andrew had been my patient and friend for many years before he had taken his new position. The dean suspected that heavy drinking was the underlying cause of Andrew's unethical behavior, which was now jeopardizing not only his career but the reputation of the medical school.

All I knew about alcoholism was what I learned in medical school, and it wasn't very much. I didn't even know what I didn't know. Nonetheless, I promised the dean that I would give Andrew a physical, a diagnosis, and the strongest possible recommendation to stop drinking.

Andrew's physical showed that he had none of the late-stage symptoms of alcoholism. He had no scarring of the liver (cirrhosis), no bleeding veins in his esophagus, no fluid accumulating in his stomach. If his face was slightly more red than usual, it was most likely from embarrassment, not from drinking too much.

Without any concrete evidence of alcoholism, I felt uncertain about how to talk with Andrew. Still, in the strongest possible terms, I advised him to quit drinking, and I suggested that he go to meetings of Alcoholics Anonymous. I also gave him a prescription for thiamine (vitamin B1), because I knew it helped to lessen the disruptions to metabolic balance caused by heavy drinking.

Andrew promised to follow my advice, and I felt quite hopeful that he could and would stop drinking. A few weeks later, he left town to give the keynote presentation at a prestigious medical conference. After his talk, Andrew skillfully fielded questions, and then went out with a colleague for "just one drink." He was completely drunk when he returned to his hotel room. Then, for reasons that he took with him to the grave, he put a bullet through his head.

Andrew's premature and senseless death shocked me. I couldn't believe that such a gifted man, so capable in every area of his life, was unable to stop drinking. Why didn't he want to quit? Why did he take his own life?

I was still pondering these mysteries when the dean of a medical school asked me to make a morning house call on a colleague, Robert, whom he suspected was drinking too much. I knew Robert by reputation as a brilliant diagnostician and researcher, and I agreed to visit him. The dean let him know we were coming.

Despite the advance notice, Robert answered the door in his underwear, carrying a large glass of whiskey in his hand. While we tried to talk with him about his drinking, he sipped from the glass and watched children's cartoons on TV. It was only when the dean threatened him with the loss of his position that he agreed to go into a treatment program.

Robert seemed to do well in treatment, but he started drinking again the minute he got home. The dean was forced to fire him, and, within a few years, Robert was dead from alcohol-related dementia. Just before he died, I saw a computerized tomography of his brain. This renowned physician had "water brain." The tissue in his brain had shrunk dramatically, and with its disappearance, the ventricles in his brain had expanded and filled with spinal fluid.

. . . . .

In the decades that followed the deaths of these two brilliant colleagues, I learned a great deal about the medical treatment of alcohol addiction. I learned about the biology of craving, and the chemical reprogramming of the brain that made addicts powerless to stop drinking. I began to understand that "alcoholic denial," the inability to recognize one's own illness, was a consequence of biological changes in the brain, not a moral failing on the part of addicted drinkers.

Along with my colleagues, I moved beyond doing mere physicals to using sophisticated assessment tools and drugs to control craving. We learned to combine the best of medical science with the insights of Alcoholics Anonymous.* In fact, we have made so much progress that today 70 percent of all physicians who enter treatment for alcoholism will recover or go "into remission."

At the same time, alcohol and drug addictions remain disorders that kill far more people than the most infectious of diseases, including the bubonic plague. Substance abuse is the elephant in the living room—and in the doctor's office. Its seemingly implacable progression causes serious emotional pain and physical disease for the family and friends of addicts. Its impact on the judgment centers of the brain has ruined the lives of millions

---

* Attendance at AA has remained a constant through the years in any good treatment program. There is now an extensive body of research that backs up the effectiveness of Twelve Step programs.

of people who have been critically injured or killed by an impaired driver. And by compromising the moral function of the brain, alcohol and drugs have enabled some of the most devastating crimes of history. Almost all war crimes are committed while under the influence.

It was my privilege as a medical doctor to spend the second half of my career studying addiction to drugs and alcohol. I headed up a major community initiative, Fighting Back, for the Robert Wood Johnson Foundation. I traveled to Russia to conduct workshops. I helped start a treatment center and a program for disruptive and misprescribing physicians. I even wrote a book, *Dying for a Drink*, with my coauthor, Barbara Thompson, to explain the medical science of addiction and recovery, including the spiritual principles of Alcoholics Anonymous.

Yet, after all these years, I find that much about this "cunning, baffling, and powerful" disease and its treatment remains a mystery, one of the most unfathomable puzzles of modern science. Drugs and alcohol have an uncanny power to ruin the lives of millions of gifted and productive people, generation after generation, in every corner of the world. Despite our tremendous advances in the neuroscience of addiction and its treatment, hardly a month goes by without someone I have known as a friend or patient dying of an alcohol-related illness or accident.

Even as I write this, I am mourning the loss of a patient, Sarah, who was an educator. Sarah took her own life because she couldn't stop drinking. Our "state-of-the-art" medical and behavioral tools were powerless in the face of the implacable progression of her illness.

In the same way that the real cause of Andrew's and Robert's deaths remained a secret, the medical examiner's report did not suggest that the cause of Sarah's death was alcoholism. In fact, today's physicians are under serious financial pressure *not* to report substance abuse as the cause of death. In most cases the hospital and the patient lose their insurance reimbursement if substance abuse is involved.

With help from medical professionals such as myself, thousands of irreplaceable and gifted individuals, like Andrew, Robert, and Sarah, are taking the secret of their addiction to the grave.

Denial

Denial is one of the great mysteries of addiction and illness in general. How can an alcoholic turning yellow from jaundice claim so convincingly that she can quit whenever she wants? Why do so many people who have had a tracheotomy for throat cancer continue to smoke through the hole in their neck? And why do even highly capable and educated people, with the first signs of cancer, put off going to the doctor until their disease has progressed to far more serious and even untreatable stages?

This all-too-human behavior as it relates to addiction is often blamed, by doctors and laypeople, on a weakness of will or general stupidity. My own guess is that the chemistry of addiction will eventually be able to explain to us the neurological mechanism of denial and even pinpoint its location in the brain. This will be a first step in developing appropriate interventions to enable addicts, at least in theory, to acknowledge their addiction and want to do something about it.

16

ANOTHER WAY FRIED CHICKEN CAN HURT YOU

Just after midnight, Jesse, a thirty-year-old woman who lived alone, came running out of her apartment screaming. A few minutes earlier, she had called me on my home phone begging for help. "It's killing me!" she said frantically. "I have a terrible pain whenever I try to go to the bathroom. It's like a knife sticking in me. Help me!"

Because Jesse lived nearby, and her pain was so acute, I agreed to make a house call. As I drove to her apartment, I reviewed the possible causes of a sudden, knifelike pain in the rectum. Thrombosis of an artery? More likely to be throbbing and slow to develop. Cancer? Also slow onset. Rectal syphilis? Most common in homosexual partners, when one partner had penile syphilis. I couldn't think of a single diagnosis that fit her symptoms.

When I saw Jesse, she was screaming under a streetlight. Clearly, there wasn't a minute to waste. I bundled her in my car, and I drove as fast as I could to the emergency room at Vanderbilt. It was just five minutes away, but Jesse's screaming made it feel like an eternity. A few blocks from the hospital, I drove the wrong way on a one-way street. Fortunately, it was the middle of the night, and there were no other cars on the road.

At the entrance to the ER, a security officer helped me carry Jesse through the door. She continued to cry and scream with pain. Nothing in my previous experience with patients had prepared me for this kind of behavior, and I remember thinking somewhat clinically that I was about to have an instructive medical experience.

I helped the nurses get Jesse up on the table, and the resident and I ordered an anuscope. This is a stainless-steel instrument for examining the rectum for a range of problems, from hemorrhoids to cancer. Word of Jesse's problem had spread, and members of the staff gathered around her bed to see if the procedure would reveal what was causing her pain.

Within minutes we could see the problem. Jesse had a small, sharp object protruding from her rectal sphincter, the muscle that helps expel or retain fecal material. With normal peristaltic movement of the bowel, excrement moves through the intestine with a series of intermittent propulsive contractions. When the rectal sphincter senses fecal material, it contracts. In Jessie's case, a sharp foreign body was stimulating the pain fibers of her rectum and causing the rectal sphincter to contract spasmodically. With every contraction, Jesse was experiencing a "knife" in her rectum.

"Have you eaten any food with bone matter in it?"

Jesse remembered eating fried chicken for dinner the previous evening. She had noticed a few small bones in a chicken leg, but they seemed insignificant, and she hadn't bothered to remove them. The resident and I looked at each other. One of those small chicken bones was lodged where it was never meant to be.

We were able to quickly anesthetize Jesse's rectal area and remove the offending sliver of bone. Jesse took a lifetime vow to be more careful when she ate fried chicken. I and the rest of the ER staff made the same promise to ourselves. Her condition illustrated a major drawback of the medical life. More and more ordinary life activities take on an ominous cast and become just one more way to end up in the emergency room.

17

JUST A QUICK QUESTION

I was standing in the food line at a church dinner, chatting with friends and noting how many of my patients were there as well. As a doctor, it's a hazard of the trade to be asked advice about physical problems in social settings, and, fairly frequently, a church member will ask me "just a quick question." Sometimes it's only the organist playing the opening hymn that saves me.

"Andy, look at my stomach." Darlene was at my elbow with her husband, Bill.* "It's suddenly swollen, and I can't get into my clothes. What causes something so strange?" Darlene turned sideways so I could get a better view. Her abdomen was clearly swollen, and I felt a chill of apprehension.

Darlene and her husband were close family friends. They had three children, and Darlene was helping to establish a children's hospital at Vanderbilt Medical Center. I had treated her once for ulcers, but she was in otherwise good health and physically fit. In the absence of overeating and overdrinking, her stomach was most likely swollen from ascites, the accumulation of fluid in the abdomen. The most common cause of this accumulation was cancer of the abdomen, liver, uterus, or ovaries.

---

* I count Bill and Darlene Hoffman among my dearest patients and friends, and Bill graciously gave permission to use their real names.

My vibrantly alive friend has advanced cancer and doesn't know it yet, I said to myself. I did not want to alarm Darlene and Bill, and I struggled to keep the anxiety and sadness out of my face.

I asked Darlene to come to my office first thing in the morning. Her exam confirmed my worst suspicions. The fluid sample from her abdomen was full of cancer cells, and she appeared to have a mass in her pelvic area. Darlene and Bill were stunned, as was I. We prayed together in my office, and I referred them to a specialist.

The oncologist assured them that there was an effective chemotherapy for Darlene's cancer, and they remained optimistic about a full recovery. Despite two years of treatment, Darlene's cancer progressed. I continued to pray with Darlene and Bill at church, with our pastor.

When Darlene was hospitalized again, I suggested to Bill that we "call the elders" for prayer, as James, the disciple of Jesus, commanded:

> *Is anyone among you sick? Then he must call the elders of the church, and they are to pray over him, anointing him with oil in the name of the Lord.*[*]

Sue and I joined other friends at a bedside gathering, and we prayed for Darlene and anointed her with oil.

Before long, it was clear that Darlene was not going to recover. She was released to hospice care, and in less than one week, she died. Bill asked me to come by their home to make one last house call for Darlene. At Darlene's bedside, I joined him and the children and the hospice nurse to whom we had grown so close. We stayed together for some time, praying and celebrating Darlene's all-too-short life. As I left, I asked Bill to call me if he needed anything.

---

* James 5:14, KJV

Six months after Darlene's death, Bill's son called to tell me that Bill wasn't doing very well. He had fallen into a deep depression after his wife's death, and he had lost interest in his work and social life. I asked Bill to come to my office for a checkup. When he arrived, his face was drawn, and there were dark circles under his eyes. He was clearly still in deep mourning for Darlene and suffering from crippling, chronic grief.

At the time, I was reading about the power of visualization for sports stars. I knew that Billie Jean King had visualized winning the U.S. Open. She saw herself standing at the net, congratulating her opponent, and accepting the trophy. With her confidence bolstered, she had won the tournament, just as she imagined.

I asked Bill if he would be willing to participate in some visualization exercises together around his grief. Because he was a devout Christian, I asked him to imagine Jesus standing at the foot of the cross. He and Darlene were to walk up to the top of the mount together. Then he would leave Darlene at the cross and walk down alone.

The following morning, Bill did the visualization by himself. Instead of walking beside Darlene, it came to him that he himself should carry his wife to the cross. "It was so perfect that it had to come from the Spirit," Bill recently wrote me. "I probably cried for an hour, but they were tears of joy. There is no doubt in my mind that this was the turning point in my recovery."

I asked Bill to come back every three weeks for a checkup, and he continued to do well. Within days, his children reported that he was eating again and seemed like his old self. Eventually, he happily remarried.

My experience with Bill was one of the most spiritually charged moments in my medical practice. Since then I have used the tool of visualization to help people cope with addiction, serious illness, anger, and a host of complicated life situations. For me it is a form of prayer to the Lord, who hears and answers prayers.

18

RHINESTONE COWBOY: ON THE BOTTLE AGAIN

When Sam Goodsong* took the stage at the Grand Ole Opry, he rocked the house. He sang of lost love, honky-tonk life, and the hardship of growing up in the mountains of East Tennessee. His beard was wild and untrimmed, and his leather boots were studded with glittering diamonds that spelled out his name. He wasn't the most famous of country music singers, but he wasn't totally second-tier, either. He produced a steady stream of good songs, and if they didn't all go gold, they made plenty of money for Sam and his producer.

As a college student occasionally hearing Sam's songs on the radio, I never dreamed that one day our paths would cross at Vanderbilt Medical Center. Sam's brother came to me on a winter afternoon to ask for help with Sam's drinking problem. Like his fans, Sam believed he wrote his best songs while drunk, but now he was drinking so much that he had been a no-show for a major concert. Sam denied that he had a drinking problem, but his brother and wife were convinced that he was drowning his talent in alcohol.

Sam's brother and I arranged to bring together the significant people in Sam's life for an intervention, a coordinated effort to convince him to enter

---

* Sam Goodsong is a composite character, representing multiple patients.

a treatment program. The intervention succeeded in part because Sam's nineteen-year-old son broke into tears. "I'm afraid you are going to die," he told his father. "I've saved you twice from choking on your own vomit."

The family loaded a still-inebriated Sam into his private jet and flew him to a treatment center, where they had prearranged for a bed. Sam was a model patient. He started to gain weight, and his memory improved. He could follow a simple conversation again. When he came back to Nashville, he was reluctant to go to AA because of his celebrity status. I convinced him that it was important, and he agreed to attend a Twelve Step meeting.

If Sam had been sick with pneumonia, most likely I would never have seen him again. But Sam had a chronic illness, addiction to alcohol, and the next time I saw him, he was drunk and lying in a hospital bed with a broken leg. He had hit another driver who was in critical condition.

Sam admitted that his craving for alcohol had returned and that he had stopped attending AA. Eventually, he had to have a drink, and once he started, he was unable to stop. He apologized in tears to his family. His wife looked down at him without a trace of pity or interest and informed him that she was getting a divorce. His son, who by then was attending Al-Anon, told his father that he was confident he could stop drinking if he returned to treatment and went back to AA.

I put Sam back on Antabuse (which would make him sick if he drank) and on a new drug that showed promise in reducing the craving for alcohol. Sam began attending meetings of AA again, and after one or two more relapses, he was able to stop drinking. His wife returned home, and his son left home to start his own family. Sam eventually went on a singing tour in the Southeast. Fortunately, his records sold reasonably well because he spent years paying off the lawsuit brought by the man he had hit while driving drunk.

Relapse

If treated properly, relapse can be a stepping-stone to a more complete recovery for an alcoholic. It underscores the importance of avoiding triggers that lead to drinking, like going back to a favorite bar, hanging out with drinking friends, and sipping small amounts of alcohol. Relapse can also lead to a renewed commitment to sobriety.

A new generation of drugs is helping alcoholics control their craving, and we are learning much more about the chemistry of addiction. Seventy years after its humble beginnings, the Twelve Traditions of Alcoholics Anonymous remain a critical tool for recovery for most alcoholics, and I always recommend it to my patients. I still on occasion attend AA meetings that are open to visitors, and I invariably experience them as a sacred place in my life, a rare venue of honest, open sharing from the depths of the human spirit.

The last time I saw Sam, he was singing a mournful tune on stage at the Grand Ole Opry. His voice had a haunting quality that I had not heard before. Perhaps his experience with death and addiction had given him the ability to appreciate his life, with all its troubles and sorrows, one day at a time. As far as I know, he never took another drink.

19

"THE ONLY SOBER PRIEST IN RUSSIA"

The alcohol consumption we have is colossal…I have been astonished to find that we drink more now than we did in the 1990s, even though those were very tough times.

—Dmitri Medvedev
President of Russia*

It was a rainy day in Moscow, in May 2001, when I pulled into the grounds of the Danilova Monastery. I had just finished attending a two-hour service in a Russian Orthodox church. Like everyone else, I had stood for the entire time, surrounded by icons and candles and children running around my legs. My spiritual reflections had been seriously limited by my strong desire to find a chair and sit down.

My host was Eugene Protsenko, the head of an alcoholism treatment center in Moscow. He was also a pioneering leader of the fledgling movement to bring Twelve Step treatment programs and Alcoholics Anonymous to Russia. I was on my second visit to Moscow since the publication of *Dying for a Drink* in Russian, and Eugene was taking me to the Danilova Monastery to meet "the only sober priest in Russia." The historic monastery

---

* *The Christian Science Monitor*, September 16, 2009

was the headquarters of the metropolitan of Moscow, the senior bishop of the Russian Church who ranked just below the patriarch.

I was looking at a white Mercedes parked outside the metropolitan's home when I noticed a man with a long white beard walking through the rain to greet us. He was dressed in a classic stovepipe hat, a long black cassock, and black boots. When he offered his hand, he introduced himself as Father Jonah, a recovering alcoholic. "I know you," he said to me. "I've read your book, *Dying for a Drink*, in Russian." It was a reminder that the world had become a very small place indeed.

Father Jonah invited us to the monastery kitchen and served us a basic Russian meal of meat and potatoes, and hard bread. Then he took us to his office in the library, where he worked as the monastery librarian. As we sat around a table surrounded by rare books and manuscripts, he explained the alcohol problems facing the Orthodox Russian Church. "Russian priests consume as much vodka as the general population and have comparably high levels of addiction," he confided.

This was unsettling news. I knew from my previous trip that four out of ten Russian men and one out of six women were alcoholics. I had also read that bootleg vodka was as cheap and accessible as bread, and half of all deaths in Russia were caused by alcohol abuse. One study showed that more Russian men had died from alcoholism than had fallen in battle during the catastrophic losses of World War II.

"The prevailing view in the church is that alcoholism is a sin," continued Father Jonah. "Addicted priests and parishioners are advised to repent and stop drinking through prayer and willpower." Since Alcoholics Anonymous was not a Christian program, the Russian Church had prohibited priests from participating in its Twelve Step program. The few priests who did get

Alcoholics Anonymous:
A Tool for Emerging Democracies

For decades, Russian doctors and psychiatrists have relied heavily on a questionable "behavior modification protocol" to treat alcoholism. Patients are injected with Antabuse or a placebo (to save money), and they are warned that drinking after an injection can result in serious illness or death. This treatment, rooted in a Pavlovian view of human nature, has been as ineffective as it is durable.

Today in Russia, Alcoholics Anonymous and Twelve Step programs are slowly gaining ground in some circles as the treatment of choice for alcoholism and drug addiction. New research suggests that Twelve Step programs have the potential not only to improve addiction recovery rates but to model democratic and egalitarian styles of group governance. This is a potentially invaluable contribution to a country suffering from centuries of autocratic leadership.*

---

* "A Russian-American Approach to the Treatment of Alcoholism in Russia: Preliminary Results," Levine, Barrett G, MD, and Ethan Nebelkopf, PhD, *Journal of Psychoactive Drugs*, 30(1): 25–32, Jan–Feb 1998

help were treated with the same ineffective medical protocols available to ordinary Russian citizens.

Father Jonah himself had tried again and again to stop drinking. In desperation and at risk to his vocation, he finally slipped away from the monastery and admitted himself to Eugene Protsenko's Twelve Step treatment program. Newly sober, he had returned to his fellow priests with a story of recovery and a copy of the Russian translation of *Dying for a Drink*.

His transformation and the moral force of his personality had convinced the metropolitan to embrace the disease model of addiction. Soon other priests were entering treatment programs and attending Alcoholics Anonymous.

"Now my dream is to visit the American treatment program run by a Catholic priest, Father Martin, so that we can create something like it here," Father Jonah added. Father Martin was a charismatic and humorous priest who had established his own treatment program in Havre de Grace, Maryland. He had also produced and starred in a series of well-known films about addiction.

Father Jonah's vision was a grand one, and I learned later that it was at least partly fulfilled. He and some colleagues were indeed sent by the metropolitan to Father Martin's training program. When they returned, they used their influence to help bring Alcoholics Anonymous to Russia and into the monastic communities to which they had given their lives.

20

WHO COULD UNDERSTAND
WHAT IT'S LIKE TO BE ME?

"I drink while I'm preparing my sermons," Rick told me. "Then I wander over to the graveyard and talk to the dead. Who else could understand what it's like to be me? I'm about to lose my wife and children *and* my vocation, and I just can't stop drinking."

Rick was the pastor of a large church, and he had just finished reading my book, *Dying for a Drink*. "My wife is driving two hours to Al-Anon in another city to keep the church from finding out. If they knew that I was an alcoholic, I'd lose my job. Can you help me?"

Coincidentally, Sue and I were flying to Rick's hometown to welcome a newly born grandchild. I agreed to see him while we were there with one condition: he would have to tell a leader in his church about his addiction and bring him or her to our meeting. Rick reluctantly agreed. A month later, with a light mist falling, we met in a private corner of a coffee shop. Rick arrived with not one but two church leaders. He had chosen wisely; both men had extensive experience working with alcohol and drug addicts.

I recommended that Rick go into treatment as soon as logistically possible. Because of his public position, I urged him to come clean with his congregation about his addiction. Their reaction and response would be out of his hands. His health and that of his family members were far more important than keeping his job. I also suggested that the men with us in the coffee shop stand with him when he made his difficult announcement.

A week later, with the two church leaders at his side, Rick announced to his congregation that he was going into treatment for alcoholism. There was a stunned silence. Then one by one, other men and women stood up in their pews to offer their support. Some went public with their own addictions. They asked Rick to return to his job when he completed his treatment program. Today, Rick is a recovering alcoholic. He is also the founder of a denomination-wide program to minister to people suffering from addiction.

The more I understand the terrible twin powers of craving and denial, the more extraordinary I find stories of recovery like Rick's. And he is not alone. Every year, men, women, and adolescents around the world begin a lifelong program of recovery or "remission" from alcohol and drug addiction. Documented rates of recovery range up to 70 percent for male physicians, in part because there are now new medications available to lessen the power of craving.[*]

As medical research advances, it also confirms the critical role of Alcoholics Anonymous and provides empirical support for some of its seemingly simple slogans. "One drink is too many, and a thousand drinks aren't enough" because alcoholism produces permanent changes in the drinker's brain. A newly sober alcoholic should attend "ninety meetings in ninety days" because it takes about three months for an addicted drinker to recover his or her cognitive capacities.

---

[*] Recovery rates go down for addicted drinkers who use drugs or have an underlying psychiatric illness, like depression, bipolar disease, or schizophrenia.

My own journey in addiction medicine came full circle when I experienced a serious emotional illness after my retirement. It had been months since I had had a good night's sleep, and I was assailed by fears, anxieties, and depression. Like Rick, I felt isolated by my sense of failure and shame, and I was convinced that no one could understand what it was like to be me.

During this time, I was working as a volunteer at a halfway house for female substance abusers. One day I took two of the staff to an Alcoholics Anonymous meeting to introduce them to the Twelve Step program. I knew the meeting was open to visitors because I had taken medical students there from my class on addiction at Vanderbilt Medical Center. As a doctor well known in the field of addiction, I had always been greeted warmly.

During the meeting, a young African American woman clearly in destitute circumstances stood up to speak. "I have to stop using pot, but I don't know how," she said. "Can anyone here help me?"

A well-dressed white woman with a refined southern accent answered her. "I can help. Marijuana is my drug of choice, too, and I know how you feel."

When I heard them speak to one another, something melted inside me. If these two women could connect so profoundly with one another, across the chasm of race and class, why couldn't I reach out for the help I needed? As much as anywhere I had ever been, this AA meeting was my spiritual home, and these were my people. I did not need to stand apart. I was no longer removed from the circle of human suffering by my career as a medical doctor and academic professor. I was just another wounded man in need of help.

When the leader asked if anyone wanted to tell something about themselves, I held up my hand. It was time to be honest. As I briefly told the story of my illness, I felt the acceptance and understanding in the room like a powerful physical presence. It was as if God's healing love itself was all around me and in me. From that day forward, I have understood what it means to be a wounded healer, to share the road to recovery with other wounded people. They walk with me, as I walk with them.

EPILOGUE

We must never put our dreams of success as God's purpose for us; God's purpose may be exactly the opposite. We have an idea that God is leading us to a particular end, a desired goal; God is not. The question of getting to a particular end is a mere incident. What we call the process, God calls the end.

—Oswald Chambers
My Utmost for His Highest

When I began my medical education in 1953, the training of doctors was based on a protocol established in 1910. We worked in a small, hierarchical team that included students, interns, nurses, and doctors. There were clear lines of authority and well-defined roles and responsibilities. If we were lucky, we had a small number of brilliant and respected mentors. Our twenty-four/seven on-call schedule enabled us to *stay with* our patients through the entire course of their illnesses, and we often developed long-term, intergenerational relationships with them and their families.

Today's generation of doctors, one of whom is my son Anderson, face far more complicated challenges. Coming of age in an era of information overload, they need to master an expanded curriculum that includes anthropology, communications, substance abuse, counseling, community-based medicine, team management, and much, much more. Of necessity, mentor-based education is giving way to an emphasis on learning how to quickly access and evaluate information from multiple sources. At the same time, the heroic and authoritative lone practitioner is being displaced by a medical team. In the course of treatment, a patient might see a primary care doctor, a nurse practitioner, a physical therapist, and multiple specialists.

For many generations of doctors, including me, it was a badge of honor to care for patients in the office *and* the hospital. It would have been unthinkable to remain in the office while a hospitalized patient reached the end of his or her life. *Staying with* a dying patient was among a doctor's most sacred responsibilities, and it could not be delegated to another. Today, for better and for worse, a patient admitted to a hospital is most likely to be cared for by a "hospitalist," a specialist whom the patient has never met before. If the patient dies in the hospital, it is this stranger, highly trained, who will be at the bedside and break the news to the family.

With the decentralization of medical care and an expanding circle of caretakers, patients gain access to deeper medical knowledge and a wider skill base. At the same time, they risk losing something of their personal relationship with a physician who feels profoundly responsible for their care—over a prolonged period of time. Team care, with its inherent danger of too many cooks in the kitchen, also creates professional rivalries and team management issues.

These problems are only compounded by the complications and irritations of managed care, with its reimbursement issues and paperwork nightmares. Doctors are forced to see more patients in less time. A doctor's treatment recommendation can be overruled by an untrained insurance employee whose eye is on the bottom line. Uninsured and underinsured patients may not be able to afford a necessary procedure or hospitalization.

"We don't have the luxury of admitting a patient to the hospital for five days to figure out what the problem is," my son Anderson tells me. His specialty, like mine, is general internal medicine. "With the pressures of contemporary medicine, it's more important than ever that medical students feel a profound sense of calling, and that they have an experience in medical school that is personally transforming."

Between the patient and the doctor lies a holy ground, for both past and present generations. I am proud to note that new generations of doctors are preserving the patient-doctor relationship as the nonnegotiable foundation of their medical practice. They are finding new ways to *stay with* their patients as they recover from illness or face impending disability or death.

Such doctors will stand on the shoulders of this passing generation of physicians as surely as we stood on the shoulders of the doctors who went before us. The stories in *Stay with Me* have been told in their honor and in honor of all the *called* physicians who will come after them.

Anderson Spickard Jr., MD

ABOUT THE AUTHORS

Anderson Spickard Jr., MD, is an Emeritus Professor of Medicine and Psychiatry at the Vanderbilt University Medical Center. He was the founding medical director of the Vanderbilt Institute for the Treatment of Addiction and the first national director of the Robert Wood Johnson Foundation's Fighting Back program, a national initiative to reduce demand for illegal drugs and alcohol. His extensive experience with patients and their families led to the publication of *Dying for a Drink: What You Should Know About Alcoholism*, coauthored with Barbara R. Thompson in 1985. The book was published in five languages and Braille, and republished in 2005.

Barbara R. Thompson is an award-winning writer, editor, and writing coach, with a focus on social issues. She has an MA in philosophy from the University of Notre Dame and has been on writing assignments to Central America, Nepal, Bangladesh, Croatia, and Bosnia. She is the cofounder of several schools for child survivors of war, including, most recently, the Global Village School of Decatur, Georgia, for unschooled teenage girls.